VEGAN COOKBOOK

LUNCH EDITION

Plant-Based Lunch Recipes with Easy Instructions

DANA TAYLOR

TABLE OF CONTENTS

TOMATO, CHICKPEA AND VEGETABLE PILAF

Healthy vegetables and pulses are the stars in this one pan wonder.

MAKES 4 SERVING/ TOTAL TIME 45 MINUTE

INGREDIENTS

1 tablespoon vegetable oil

1 medium brown onion, chopped

1 tablespoon korma curry paste

1 1/4 cups basmati rice, rinsed

2 cups Massel vegetable liquid stock

400g can diced tomatoes

250g cauliflower, cut into florets

400g can chickpeas, drained, rinsed

50g baby spinach

1 tablespoon finely chopped fresh coriander leaves

METHOD

STEP 1

Heat oil in a large, heavy-based saucepan over medium heat. Add onion. Cook, stirring occasionally, for 4 to 5 minutes or until onion is tender. Add curry paste. Cook, stirring, for 1 minute or until fragrant.

STEP 2

Add rice, stock, tomato and cauliflower. Increase heat to high. Bring to the boil. Reduce heat to low. Simmer, covered, for 15 to 17 minutes or until rice is tender and liquid has absorbed.

STEP 3

Add chickpeas, spinach and coriander. Season with pepper. Stir to combine. Stand, covered, for 5 minutes. Serve.

NUTRITION VALUE

1698 KJ Energy, 8g fat, 1g saturated fat, 7g fiber, 12g protein, 66g carbs.

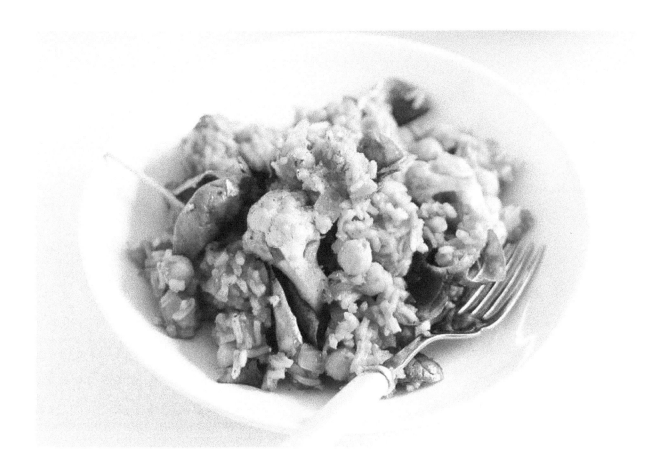

HEALTHY FRIED RICE

This **vegetarian** version of traditional fried rice is lower in kilojoules but full of flavor.

MAKES 4 SERVING/ TOTAL TIME 20 MINUTE

INGREDIENTS

2 teaspoons sesame oil

1/2 Chinese cabbage, shredded

1 carrot, cut into matchsticks

1 small red capsicum, seeds removed, sliced

3 cups cooked brown rice

2 tablespoons light soy sauce

2 tablespoons ketjap manis*, plus extra to drizzle

1/2 cup cashew nuts, lightly toasted

6 spring onions, thinly sliced on the diagonal

METHOD

STEP 1

Heat oil in a large wok over high heat. Add cabbage, carrot and capsicum, and stir-fry for 1-2 minutes.

STEP 2

Add rice and cook for a further 2 minutes. Add soy, ketjap manis, cashews and half the spring onions, toss to combine.

STEP 3

To serve, garnish with remaining onions and drizzle with extra ketjap manis.

NUTRITION VALUE

1549 KJ Energy, 13g fat, 2g saturated fat, 9g protein, 51g carbs.

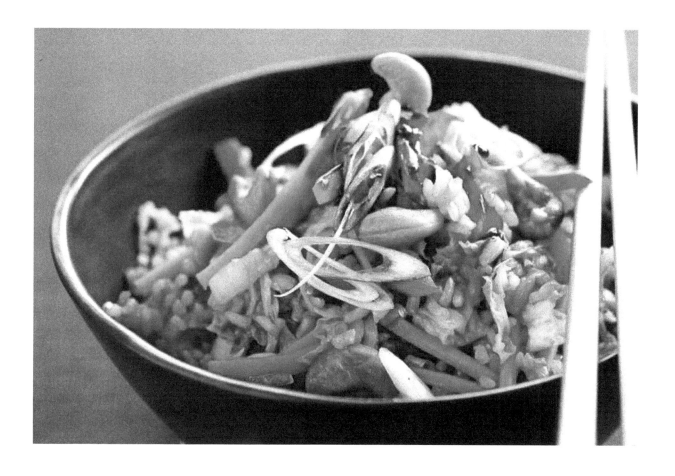

FUSILLI WITH ROASTED VEGETABLES AND BASIL PESTO

Meat-free Monday just became more exciting with this versatile **vegetarian** pasta.

MAKES 4 SERVING/ TOTAL TIME 50 MINUTE

INGREDIENTS

350g jap pumpkin, peeled

1 small sweet potato, peeled

2 carrots, peeled

2 zucchinis, trimmed

4 yellow squash, trimmed

2 tablespoons olive oil

500g dried fusilli pasta

BASIL PESTO

1 1/2 cups (firmly packed) fresh basil leaves

1/2 cup pine nuts

2 garlic cloves, roughly chopped

1/2 cup extra-virgin olive oil

60g parmesan cheese (or vegetarian hard cheese), finely grated

METHOD

STEP 1

Preheat oven to 200°C. Line 2 baking trays with baking paper. Cut pumpkin, sweet potato, carrots, zucchinis and squash into 2cm cubes. Place vegetables in a large bowl. Add oil and season with salt and pepper. Toss to coat. Spread on prepared baking trays. Roast for 40 minutes, swapping trays around in oven after 20 minutes, or until golden and tender.

STEP 2

Meanwhile, make pesto: Place basil, pine nuts and garlic in a food processor. Process until almost smooth. With the motor running, add oil in a slow and steady stream. Process until all oil is combined. Transfer pesto to a bowl. Add parmesan. Season with salt and pepper. Stir until well combined.

STEP 3

Return pasta to saucepan over low heat. Add roasted vegetables. Toss until well combined. Season with salt and pepper. Spoon into bowls. Top with 1/3 cup pesto and serve.

NUTRITION VALUE

2939 KJ Energy, 21g fat, 4g saturated fat, 9g fiber, 20g protein, 105g carbs.

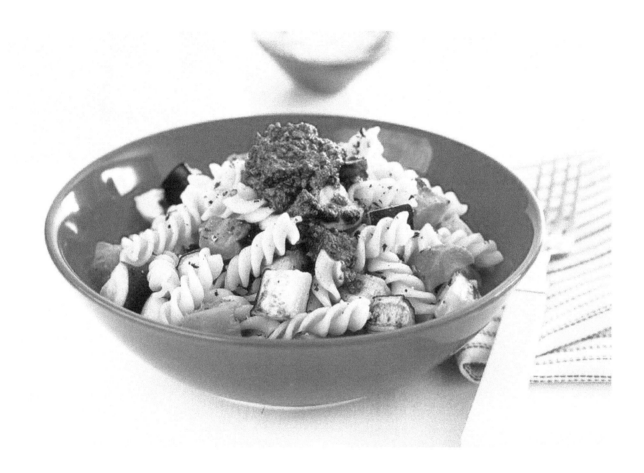

VEGETABLE SUNG CHOI BAO

Recipe that everyone loves!

MAKES 4 SERVING/ TOTAL TIME 15 MINUTE

INGREDIENTS

1 425g can young corn cuts, drained

1 280g can mushrooms, drained

1 230g can water chestnuts, drained

3 green shallots, trimmed, chopped

2 teaspoons olive oil

1 garlic clove, crushed

3 teaspoons soy sauce

1 teaspoon finely chopped fresh ginger

4 whole iceberg lettuce inner leaves, washed, dried

Coriander leaves, to serve

METHOD

STEP 1

Place the corn, mushrooms, water chestnuts and green shallots in the bowl of a food processor. Process until roughly chopped.

STEP 2

Heat the oil in a wok or medium non-stick frying pan over medium-high heat. Add the vegetable mixture, garlic, soy sauce and ginger, and stir-fry for 2-3 minutes or until heated through.

STEP 3

Divide the mixture among the lettuce cups. Sprinkle with the coriander leaves and serve immediately.

NUTRITION VALUE

223 KJ Energy, 3g fat,
6g fiber, 3g protein, 2g carbs.

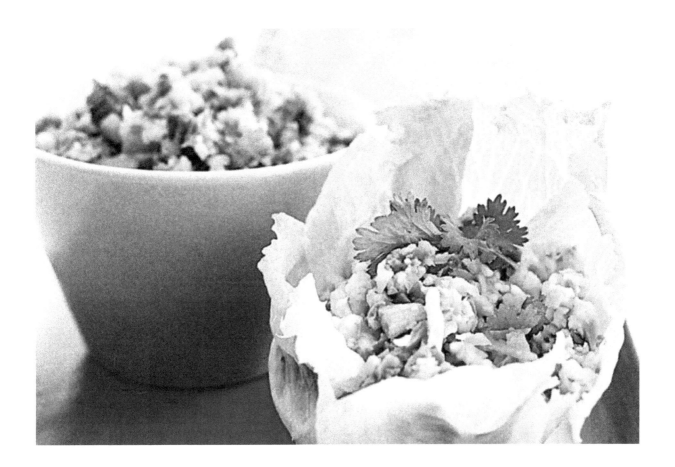

TOFU & PUMPKIN GREEN CURRY

Feed the family with this hearty **vegetarian** curry served with flavorsome sesame brown rice.

MAKES 4 SERVING/ TOTAL TIME 30 MINUTE

INGREDIENTS

1 tablespoon vegetable oil

1 x 300g pkt firm tofu, drained, thickly sliced crossways

1 x 270ml can light coconut milk

125ml (1/2 cup) water

2 tablespoons green curry paste

600g Kent pumpkin, deseeded, peeled, cut into 3cm pieces

250g green beans, topped

3 teaspoons brown sugar

1 1/2 tablespoons fresh lime juice

1/2 cup fresh coriander leaves, to serve

SESAME BROWN RICE

2 tablespoons sesame seeds

750ml (3 cups) water

360g (3 cups) long-grain brown rice

METHOD

STEP 1

Heat a medium saucepan over medium heat. Add the sesame seeds and cook, tossing, for 1 minute or until lightly toasted.

STEP 2

Add the water. Add rice and bring back to the boil. Reduce heat to medium-low and simmer, slightly covered, for 10 minutes , Add the tofu and cook for 3-4 minutes each side or until golden. Transfer to a plate.

STEP 3

Add the coconut milk, water and curry paste to the pan and cook, stirring, for 1 minute. Add the pumpkin. Add the beans and cook, covered, for 5 minutes or until the pumpkin is tender and the beans are bright green and tender crisp. Add the sugar and lime juice.

Step 4

Add to the curry and gently stir until just heated through. Spoon the sesame brown rice among serving bowls. Top with the curry

NUTRITION VALUE	950 KJ Energy, 11g fat, 3.5g saturated fat, 6g fiber, 12g protein, 19g carbs.

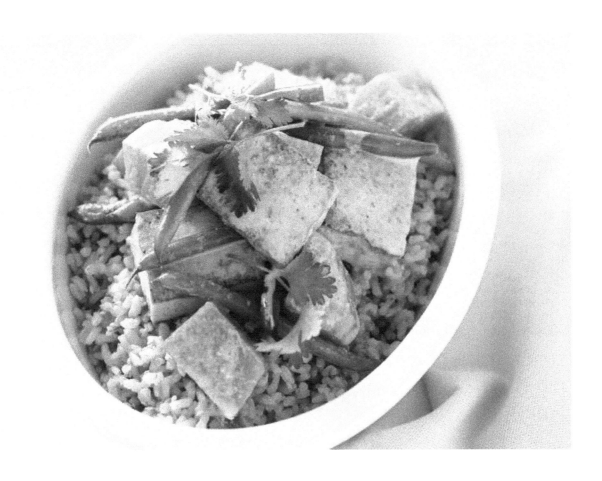

RED LENTIL AND SPINACH DHAL

Try your hand at an Indian dhal!

MAKES 4 SERVING/ TOTAL TIME 50 MINUTE

INGREDIENTS

1 tablespoon peanut oil

2 medium brown onions, thinly sliced

1 garlic clove, crushed

1 tablespoon ground coriander

1 teaspoon ground cumin

1 teaspoon ground turmeric

2 cups red lentils

400g can crushed tomatoes

50g baby spinach, trimmed, chopped

1/3 cup fresh coriander leaves

4 chapatti breads, warmed

METHOD

STEP 1

Heat oil in a saucepan over medium heat. Add onion. Cook, stirring, for 5 minutes or until soft. Add garlic, coriander, cumin and turmeric. Cook, stirring, for 1 minute or until fragrant.

STEP 2

Add lentils, tomato and 2 1/2 cups cold water. Cover. Bring to the boil. Reduce heat to low. Simmer, stirring occasionally, for 20 minutes or until lentils are tender. Add spinach. Cook, stirring, for 2 minutes or until spinach is wilted.

STEP 3

Top lentil mixture with coriander. Season with pepper. Serve with chapatti bread.

NUTRITION VALUE

1794 KJ Energy, 8g fat, 1g saturated fat, 19g fiber, 28g protein, 52g carbs.

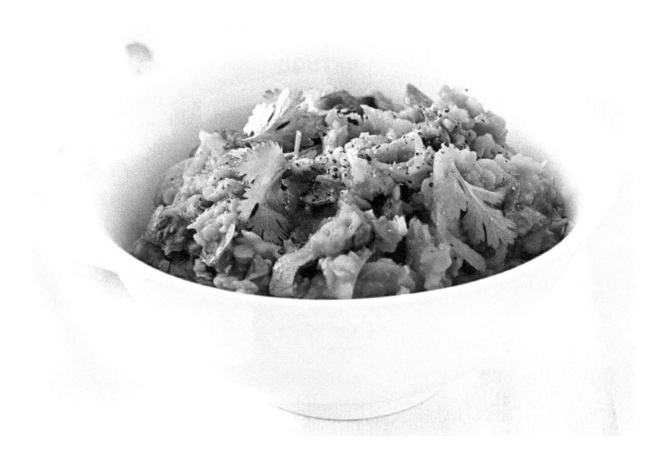

ROASTED PUMPKIN AND CHICKPEA SALAD

Serve up an impressive roasted pumpkin and chickpea salad for Meat-free Monday.

MAKES 8 SERVING/ TOTAL TIME 40 MINUTE

INGREDIENTS

1.2kg Jap pumpkin, peeled, deseeded, cut into 1cm-thick wedges

3 teaspoons caster sugar

2 tablespoons olive oil

2 x 400g cans chickpeas, drained, rinsed

75g toasted slivered almonds

1/3 cup white balsamic vinegar

3 garlic cloves, crushed

1 lemon, rind finely grated

1 cup flat-leaf parsley leaves

METHOD

STEP 1

Preheat oven to 220°C. Divide pumpkin between 2 large baking trays. Season with salt and pepper. Sprinkle with sugar and drizzle with oil. Roast for 30 to 40 minutes, swapping trays after 20 minutes, or until golden and tender. Set aside to cool.

STEP 2

Place pumpkin on a large plate. Add chickpeas and almonds. Toss to combine. Cover and refrigerate until required.

STEP 3

Whisk vinegar, garlic and lemon rind in a jug. Season with salt and pepper. Pour dressing over pumpkin salad. Sprinkle with parsley. Toss gently to combine. Serve.

NUTRITION VALUE

983 KJ Energy, 11g fat, 1g saturated fat, 9g protein, 21g carbs.

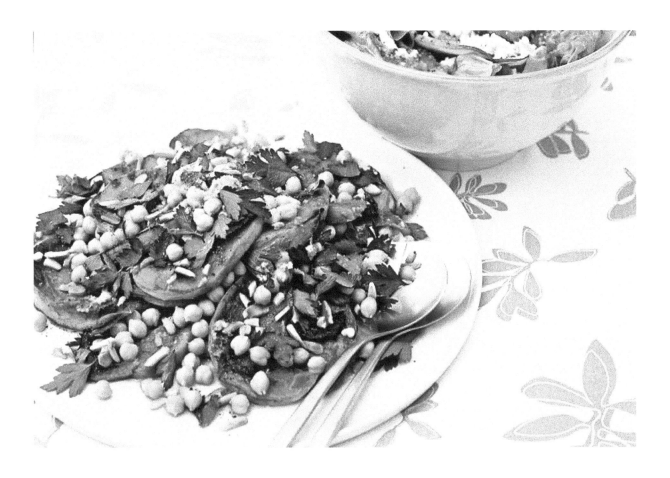

PUMPKIN AND GREEN BEAN PILAF

Looking for a new way to serve rice and vegies? Try this!

MAKES 4 SERVING/ TOTAL TIME 30 MINUTE

INGREDIENTS

300g (1 1/2 cups) white long-grain rice

1L (4 cups) Massel vegetable liquid stock

500g butternut pumpkin, deseeded, peeled, cut into 2cm pieces

1 teaspoon ground cumin

200g green beans, topped, cut into 6cm pieces

45g (1/4 cup) pine nuts

1 tablespoon olive oil

1 red onion, halved, thinly sliced

1/4 cup loosely packed fresh continental parsley leaves

METHOD

STEP 1

Combine rice, stock, pumpkin and cumin in a large saucepan. Cover and bring to the boil over high heat. Reduce heat to medium and cook, covered, for 12 minutes or until rice and pumpkin are tender. Add the beans 2 minutes before the end of cooking. Remove from heat. Cover and set aside for 5 minutes or until all the liquid is absorbed.

STEP 2

Meanwhile, heat a non-stick frying pan over medium-high heat. Add the pine nuts and cook, stirring, for 2 minutes or until toasted. Transfer to a bowl. Heat the oil in the same pan over medium heat. Add the onion and cook, stirring, for 6 minutes or until brown. Remove from heat.

STEP 3

Spoon the pilaf among serving bowls. Top with fried onion, and sprinkle with toasted pine nuts and parsley.

NUTRITION VALUE

2054 KJ Energy, 15g fat, 2g saturated fat, 5g fiber, 13g protein, 72g carbs.

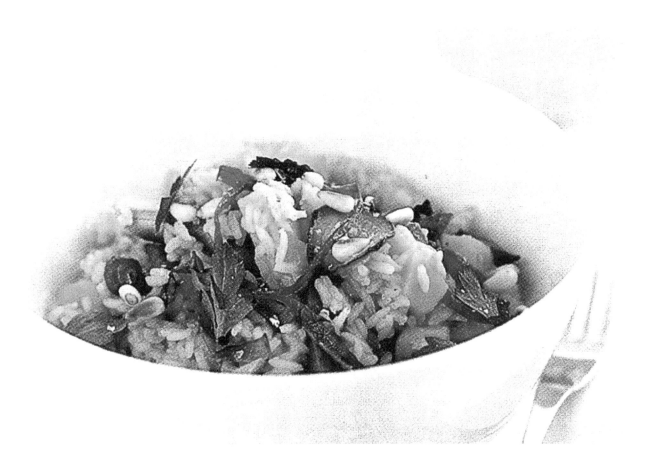

HERBED RICE SALAD

Add flavor to tonight's rice dish with this beautiful flavor combination of sweet currants and crunchy almonds.

MAKES 8 SERVING/ TOTAL TIME 60 MINUTE

INGREDIENTS

1.25L (5 cups) water

400g (2 cups) long-grain brown rice

50g (1/3 cup) slivered almonds

55g (1/3 cup) currants

1/3 cup loosely packed coarsely chopped fresh continental parsley

1/3 cup loosely packed coarsely chopped fresh coriander

2 1/5 tablespoons fresh lemon juice

1 tablespoon olive oil

Freshly ground black pepper

METHOD

STEP 1

Place water in a saucepan over low heat. Stir in rice and simmer, covered, for 45-50 minutes or until water is absorbed and rice is tender. Remove from heat. Transfer to a large heatproof bowl.

STEP 2

Meanwhile, place the almonds in a non-stick frying pan over medium heat. Cook, stirring, for 1-2 minutes or until toasted. Remove from heat. Add the almonds, currants, parsley and coriander to the rice and gently toss to combine.

STEP 3

Whisk together the lemon juice and oil in a small bowl. Season with pepper. Add dressing to the rice and toss to coat. Serve.

NUTRITION VALUE

915 KJ Energy, 6.5g fat, 1g saturated fat, 2.5g fiber, 4g protein, 37g carbs.

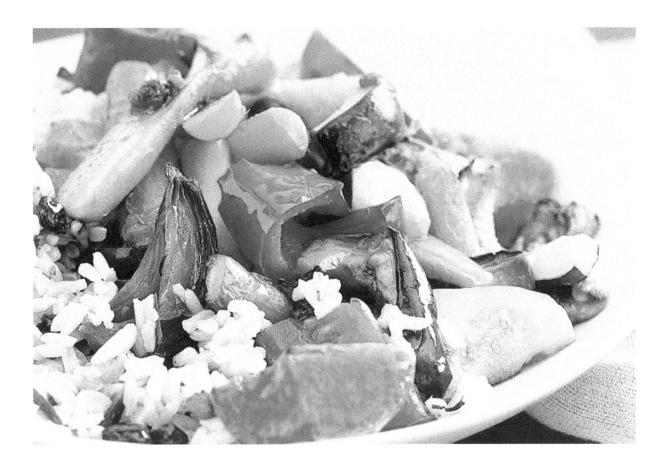

JAPANESE TOFU WITH ASIAN GREENS SALAD

Mouth-watering Asian greens combine with the golden tofu to create an elegant side dish.

MAKES 4 SERVING/ TOTAL TIME 14 MINUTE

INGREDIENTS

80ml (1/3 cup) vegetable oil

1 x 200g pkt Japanese tofu drained, cut into 2cm cubes

1 x 100g pkt baby Asian greens

85g (1 1/4 cups) bean sprouts

1 1/2 kecap manis

METHOD

STEP 1

Heat 1 tablespoon of the oil in a medium non-stick frying pan over high heat. Add the tofu and cook for 2 minutes each side or until golden. Transfer to a plate lined with paper towel.

STEP 2

Divide baby Asian greens among serving plates. Top with the bean sprouts and tofu. Place the remaining oil and kecap manis in a small screw-top jar and shake until well combined. Drizzle salad and tofu with dressing and serve immediately.

NUTRITION VALUE

1140 KJ Energy, 24g fat, 2.5g saturated fat, 1.5g fiber, 11g protein, 4.5g carbs.

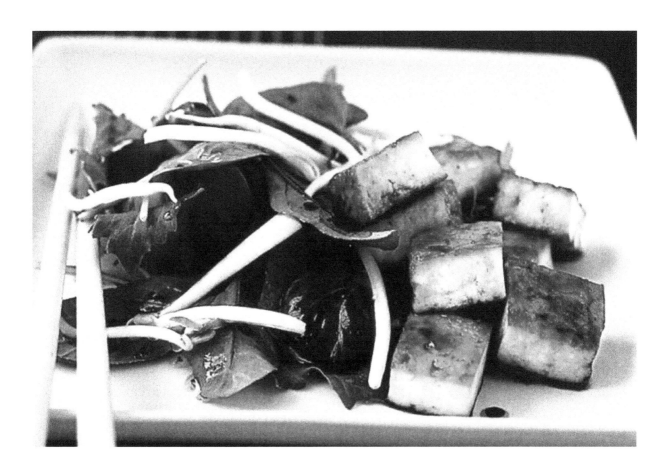

ROLLINI WITH SEMI-DRIED TOMATOES

Recipe that everyone loves!

MAKES 4 SERVING/ TOTAL TIME 35 MINUTE

INGREDIENTS

500g eggplant, cut into 2cm cubes

1/3 cup olive oil

500g San Remo Rollini pasta

1/4 cup balsamic vinegar

1 teaspoon Dijon mustard

1 cup semi-dried tomatoes, chopped

1/4 cup fresh oregano leaves

METHOD

STEP 1

Preheat oven to 200°C. Line a tray with baking paper. Place eggplant onto tray. Drizzle with 2 tablespoons of oil. Season. Roast for 20 minutes, or until tender.

STEP 2

Cook pasta following packet directions.

STEP 3

Whisk vinegar, mustard, remaining oil, and salt and pepper in a jug to combine.

STEP 4

Drain pasta, reserving 2 tablespoons of cooking water. Return pasta and water to saucepan. Add eggplant, vinegar mixture, tomatoes and oregano. Toss over low heat until well combined. Serve.

NUTRITION VALUE

3070 KJ Energy, 24g fat, 4g saturated fat, 21g protein, 102g carbs.

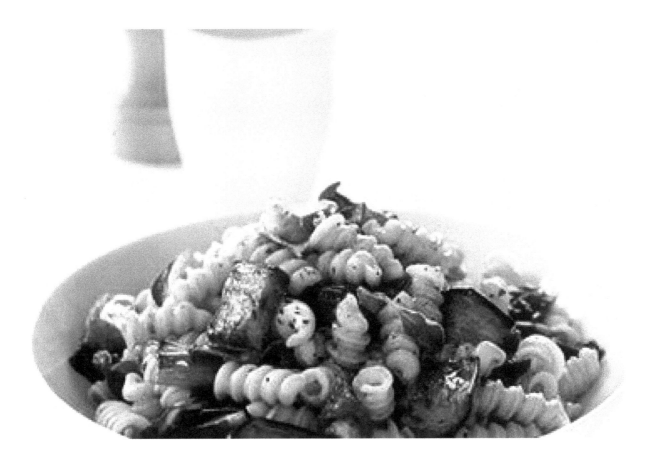

ROASTED BEETROOT, SWEET POTATO AND COUSCOUS SALAD

Try this fast, fresh and fabulous dish and see for yourself!

MAKES 4 SERVING/ TOTAL TIME 50 MINUTE

INGREDIENTS

1 bunch beetroot, trimmed, peeled, cut into thin wedges

500g orange sweet potato, peeled, cut into 2cm pieces

1 tablespoon olive oil

1 1/4 cups couscous

50g baby rocket

1/3 cup French dressing

METHOD

STEP 1

Preheat oven to 240C/220C fan-forced. Line a large baking tray with baking paper. Arrange beetroot on 1 half of prepared tray. Place sweet potato on remaining half. Drizzle with oil. Bake for 25 minutes or until golden and tender.

STEP 2

Meanwhile, place couscous in a large, heatproof bowl. Add 1 1/4 cups boiling water. Cover. Stand for 5 minutes. Stir with a fork to separate grains. Add beetroot, sweet potato, rocket and dressing. Toss to combine. Season with salt and pepper. Serve.

NUTRITION VALUE

1746 KJ Energy, 8g fat, 1g saturated fat, 5.8g fiber, 11.8g protein, 70.9g carbs.

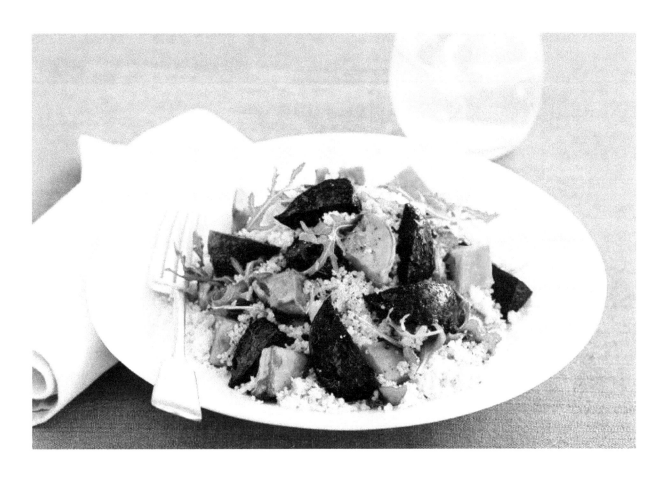

SEARED CHILLI TOFU WITH ASIAN GREENS

A tasty **vegetarian** meal, prepared in a flash using healthy ingredients such as tofu, Asian greens and chili.

MAKES 4 SERVING/ TOTAL TIME 20 MINUTE

INGREDIENTS

1 x 350g pkt firm tofu

2 tablespoons soy sauce

2 teaspoons canola oil

1 garlic clove, crushed

1 teaspoon finely chopped fresh red chili

1 bunch gai larn, trimmed, washed, dried

1 bunch choy sum, trimmed, washed, dried

750ml (3 cups) Massel vegetable liquid stock

750ml (3 cups) water

1 teaspoon sesame oil

1 tablespoon kecap manis

METHOD

STEP 1

Cut the tofu crossways into quarters. Pat dry both sides of tofu squares with paper towel. Combine the soy sauce, canola oil, garlic and chili in a small bowl. Turn to coat. Cover with plastic wrap and place in the fridge for 1 hour to develop the flavors. Cut the stems from the leaves of the gai larn and choy sum. Place the stock and water in a large saucepan over high heat. Bring to the boil. Add the gai larn and choy sum stems, cover, and return to the boil. Cook, covered, for 2 minutes or until bright green and tender crisp Add the gai larn and choy sum leaves to the pan and cook, covered, for 1 minute .

STEP 2

Meanwhile, drain the tofu and discard the marinade. Heat the sesame oil in a large non-stick frying pan over medium-high heat. Add the tofu and kecap manis and cook for 1-2 minutes each side or until tofu is golden brown. Divide Asian greens among plates. Top with tofu and serve immediately.

NUTRITION VALUE

1070 KJ Energy, 14g fat, 1.5g saturated fat, 3.5g fiber, 19g protein, 15g carbs.

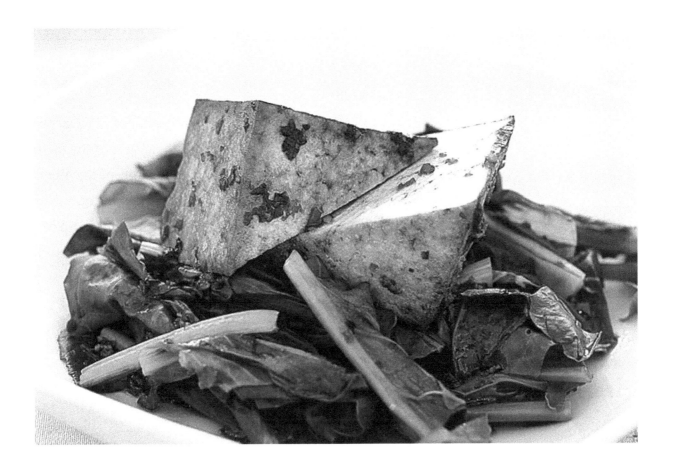

ROSEMARY & POTATO BREAD

Recipe that everyone loves!

MAKES 6 SERVING/ TOTAL TIME 60 MINUTE

INGREDIENTS

600g (4 cups) plain flour, sifted

1 tablespoon (14g/2 sachets) dried yeast

2 teaspoons salt

2 teaspoons finely chopped fresh rosemary leaves

310ml (1 1/4 cups) warm water

5 tablespoons olive oil

Olive oil, to grease

2 medium desiree or pontiac potatoes, unpeeled

10 x 3cm-long fresh rosemary sprigs

2 teaspoons sea salt flakes

METHOD

STEP 1

Place the flour, yeast, salt and rosemary in a large bowl and mix well. Make a well in the center of the mixture. Combine the water and 3 tablespoons of the oil and add to the dry ingredients. together. Turn the dough onto a lightly oiled surface and knead in 1 tablespoon of remaining oil. Knead for 10 minutes or until smooth and elastic. Brush a large bowl with oil to grease. Place the dough in the bowl and turn to coat with oil. Cover with a clean tea towel and place in a warm, draught-free place to prove for 45 minutes or until the dough doubles in size. Preheat oven to 220°C. Without knocking back (deflating) the dough, place in a 15 x 27cm non-stick loaf pan.

STEP 2

Cut the potatoes, Drizzle with the remaining oil and toss to coat. Use a small, sharp knife to cut 20 evenly spaced slits, about 2cm deep and 2cm long, in the top of the dough. Insert 1 slice of potato in each and insert a rosemary sprig in the dough between the potato slices. Sprinkle the top of the dough with sea salt and bake in a preheated oven for 40 minutes Serve warm or at room temperature.

NUTRITION VALUE

2220 KJ Energy, 16g fat, 3g saturated fat, 13g protein, 79g carbs.

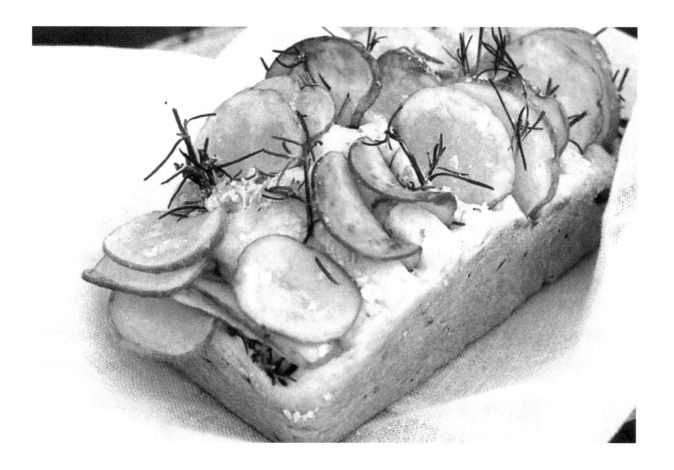

BEAN AND ROCKET SALAD WITH GREEN-OLIVE DRESSING

Whip up this healthy green salad in a flash - its nutritious and full of flavor!

MAKES 6 SERVING/ TOTAL TIME 15 MINUTE

INGREDIENTS

200g green beans, topped, cut into 3cm lengths

100g baby rocket leaves

GREEN-OLIVE DRESSING

100g drained green olives, pitted, finely chopped

60ml (1/4 cup) olive oil

2 tablespoons balsamic vinegar

1 tablespoon seeded mustard

Salt & freshly ground black pepper

METHOD

STEP 1

To make the dressing, combine olives, oil, vinegar and mustard in a screw-top jar and shake well until combined. Taste and season with salt and pepper.

STEP 2

Cook beans in a medium saucepan of salted boiling water for 5 minutes or until bright green and tender crisp. Drain. Refresh under cold running water. Drain.

STEP 3

Place rocket and beans in a serving bowl. Drizzle with green-olive dressing and toss to combine. Serve immediately.

NUTRITION VALUE

1190 KJ Energy, 8.7g fat, 1.9g saturated fat, 13.6g fiber, 11.3g protein, 32.2g carbs.

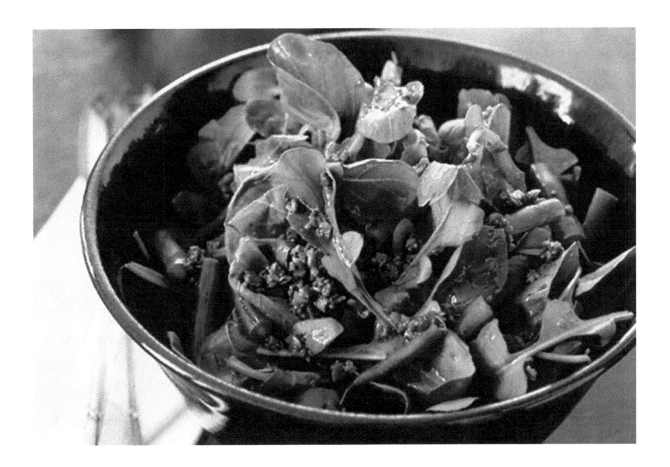

HASH BROWNS WITH BABY TOMATOES AND SPINACH

Recipe that everyone loves!

MAKES 4 SERVING/ TOTAL TIME 60 MINUTE

INGREDIENTS

250g cherry truss tomatoes

Olive oil spray

4 large sebago potatoes

1/3 cup (80ml) olive oil

150g baby spinach leaves

METHOD

STEP 1

Preheat oven to 200°C. Use scissors to remove the tomatoes from the truss, leaving the tops intact. Place the tomatoes on a baking tray. Spray lightly with the olive oil. Roast for 15-20 minutes , Meanwhile, peel and coarsely grate the potatoes. Squeeze handfuls of the grated potato to remove as much liquid as possible. Place the grated potato into a large bowl.

STEP 2

Heat half the oil in a large non-stick frying pan over a medium-high heat. Place 1/4 cup of the grated potato in the pan. Use an egg flip to flatten slightly to form a 10cm round. Repeat to make three more. Cook for 2-3 minutes each side or until golden. Transfer to a plate. Cover with foil. Repeat with the remaining potato.

STEP 3

Heat a frying pan or saucepan over a medium-high heat. Wash the spinach and add to the pan and cook for 1-2 minutes or until wilted. Serve hash browns topped with the spinach and tomatoes.

NUTRITION VALUE

1229 KJ Energy, 18g fat, 3g saturated fat, 6g protein, 24g carbs.

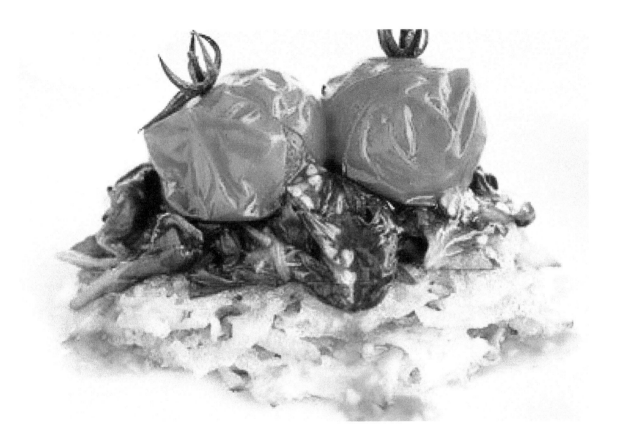

BARBEQUED MUSHROOM AND PUMPKIN SALAD

This **vegan** pumpkin salad is full of healthy vegetables and tantalizing spices.

MAKES 4 SERVING/ TOTAL TIME 23 MINUTE

INGREDIENTS

1kg pumpkin, cut into 1cm-thick wedges

6 flat mushrooms, sliced

1/2 cup (125ml) olive oil

2 tablespoons brown sugar

2 teaspoons ground cumin

Salt & freshly ground pepper

2 tablespoons fresh lemon juice

160g baby spinach leaves

Crusty bread, to serve

METHOD

STEP 1

Place 1/2 the pumpkin in a single layer onto a microwave safe plate. Cover and microwave on High for 4 minutes. Repeat with remaining pumpkin. Set aside for 5 minutes.

STEP 2

Place mushrooms in a shallow dish. Combine 1/4 cup (60ml) olive oil, brown sugar, cumin and salt and pepper in a screw-top jar and shake well to combine. Pour the dressing over the mushrooms, toss well. Cover and set aside 5 minutes.

STEP 3

Combine the remaining olive oil, lemon juice, salt and pepper in a screw-top jar, shake well to combine.

STEP 4

Preheat a barbeque plate on a medium-high heat. Add the mushrooms and cook, tossing frequently, for 2-3 minutes. Transfer to a plate. Add the pumpkin and cook 2-3 minutes each side. Arrange the spinach, mushrooms and pumpkin onto serving plate. Drizzle dressing. Serve with bread.

NUTRITION VALUE	1658 KJ Energy, 29g fat, 5g saturated fat, 8g fiber, 5g protein, 24g carbs.

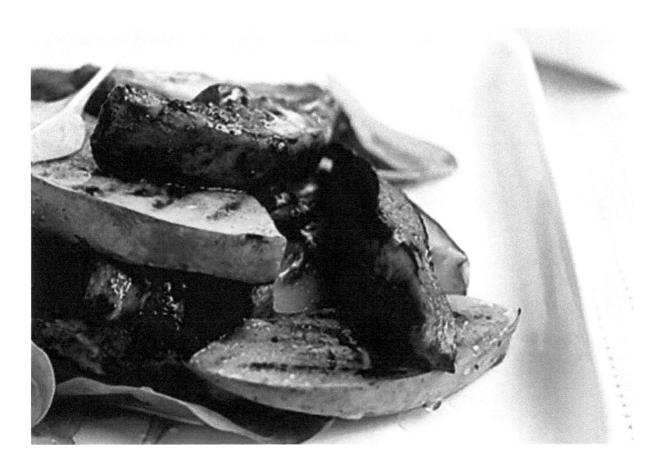

SPICED ONION NAAN WITH LENTIL SALAD

Recipe that everyone loves!

MAKES 2 SERVING/ TOTAL TIME 30 MINUTE

INGREDIENTS

1/4 cup (60ml) olive oil

2 onions, thinly sliced

2 teaspoons curry powder

2 naan bread*

50g grated cheddar

1 garlic clove, finely chopped

1 tablespoon lemon juice, plus wedges to serve

120g baby spinach leaves

2 x 400g cans brown lentils, rinsed, drained

METHOD

STEP 1

Preheat the oven to 180°C and lightly grease a baking tray.

STEP 2

Heat half the oil in a large pan on medium-low heat. Add onion and cook, stirring, for 8-10 minutes until soft and tinged golden. Add 1 1/2 teaspoons curry powder, and then stir for 1 minute. Remove from heat.

STEP 3

Place naan on a baking tray, sprinkle with cheese and top with three-quarters of the onion. Bake for 5-6 minutes until golden brown and cheese has melted.

STEP 4

Meanwhile, whisk remaining oil and curry with garlic, juice, salt and pepper in a bowl. Add remaining onion, spinach and lentils. Toss to combine. Serve with naan.

NUTRITION VALUE

3570 KJ Energy, 46g fat, 12g saturated fat, 15g fiber, 34g protein, 70g carbs.

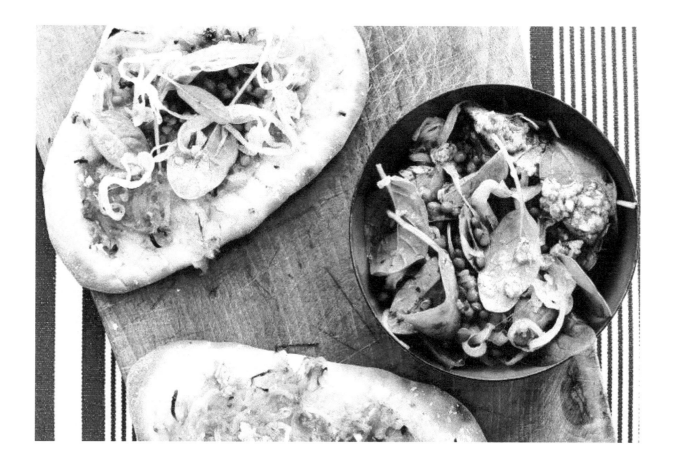

VEGETARIAN CHILLI

Lentils and beans make this vegetarian chili extra hearty and filling.

MAKES 4 SERVING/ TOTAL TIME 35 MINUTE

INGREDIENTS

80ml (1/3 cup) olive oil

1 large onion, peeled, finely chopped

1 small red chili, seeded, chopped

1/2 red capsicum, chopped

1/4 teaspoon chili flakes

1/2 teaspoon ground cinnamon

1 teaspoon ground cumin

1 teaspoon dried thyme

2-3 garlic cloves, crushed

420g can mixed beans, drained, rinsed

420g can lentils, drained, rinsed

425g can diced tomatoes

1 tablespoon tomato paste

1 cup chopped flat-leaf parsley

METHOD

STEP 1

Place 2 tablespoons of oil in a large saucepan over medium heat. Add the onion, fresh chili and capsicum and cook until softened. Add the chili flakes, cinnamon, cumin and thyme and cook for a further minute.

STEP 2

Reduce heat to low and add the garlic, beans, lentils, tomatoes, tomato paste and remaining oil.

STEP 3

Cover and simmer for 15 minutes, stirring occasionally. Remove lid and cook for a further 5 minutes or until thickened.

STEP 4

Stir through the parsley and serve with warm flour tortillas or steamed rice and sprinkled with grated cheese, if desired.

NUTRITION VALUE

2299 KJ Energy, 49g fat, 7g saturated fat, 11g fiber, 9g protein, 16g carbs.

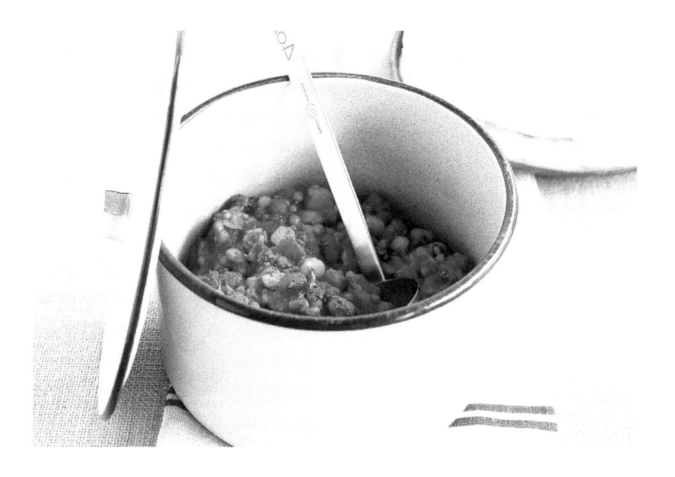

SPICY ROASTED CAULIFLOWER RECIPE

Roasted cauliflower is a fast and easy recipe that turns this unassuming and healthy vegetable into a star

MAKES 4 SERVING/ TOTAL TIME 35 MINUTE

INGREDIENTS

teaspoon smoked paprika

¼ teaspoon turmeric

½ teaspoon garlic powder

½ teaspoon freshly ground black pepper

½ teaspoon fine sea salt

1 head cauliflower - cut into florets

3 tablespoons extra-virgin olive oil

Fresh parsley - chopped

METHOD

STEP 1

Adjust the oven rack to the middle position, and preheat oven to 425°F.

In a small bowl, add smoked paprika, turmeric, garlic powder salt and black pepper. Mix everything very well.

STEP 2

Place the cauliflower florets on an aluminum foil lined baking sheet. Pour olive oil on top of the cauliflower florets and toss until everything is evenly coated.

Sprinkle the spice mixture over the cauliflower, and mix well to combine.

Roast for about 25-30 minutes or until the cauliflower is tender and golden brown

Garnish with fresh parsley. Enjoy!

NUTRITION VALUE

111 Energy, 10.6g fat, 1.5g saturated fat, 1.9g fiber, 1.5g protein, 4.4g carbs.

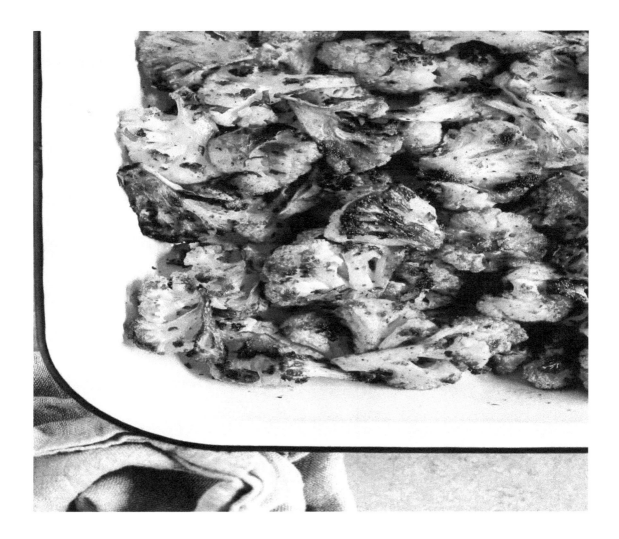

EASY ZUCCHINIS CAULIFLOWER RICE

Cauliflower rice is a quick and easy way to replace starchy rice in any dish.

MAKES 4 SERVING/ TOTAL TIME 10 MINUTE

INGREDIENTS

2 tbsp - olive oil

1 cup red onions - chopped

2 cups zucchinis - diced

1/2 tsp garlic powder

salt and black pepper to taste

5 cups cauliflower - cut into small florets

1 ½ tablespoon pesto

1 tbsp hemp seeds

Fresh parsley for garnishing - chopped

METHOD

STEP 1

Pulse the cauliflower florets in a food processor for about 25-30 seconds until it's a rice-like consistency. Set aside.

STEP 2

Add oil on pot or skillet over medium heat. Sauté onion for about 5 minutes. Then add zucchinis, garlic powder, salt and black pepper. Cook for about 4 minutes.

Add riced cauliflower and mix everything well. Cook until tender.

When it's time to serve, top with hemp seeds and fresh chopped parsley.

NUTRITION VALUE

180 Energy, 13g fat, 2g saturated fat, 4g fiber, 5g protein, 10g carbs.

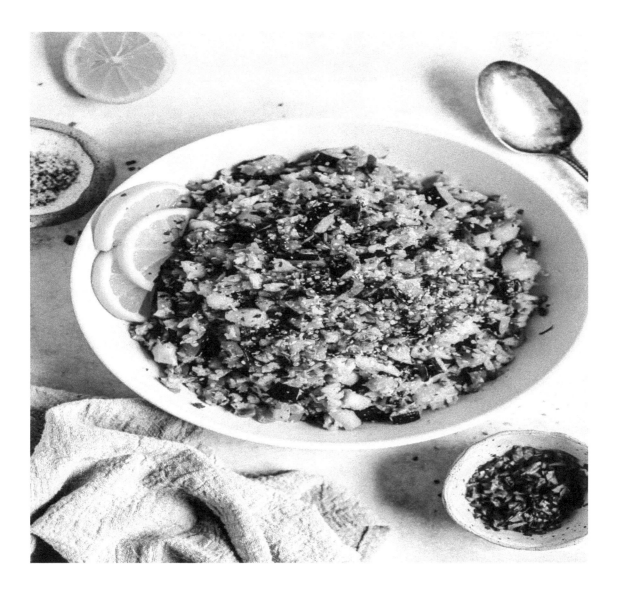

ROASTED BUTTERNUT SQUASH RECIPE

Roasted butternut squash is a delicious and healthy side dish recipe to make for lunch and dinner and serve with beef, chicken and fish.

MAKES 6 SERVING/ TOTAL TIME 20 MINUTE

INGREDIENTS

3 lb. butternut squash

2 tbsp olive oil

1/2 tsp salt

1/4 tsp black pepper

½ tsp paprika

Fresh parsley to taste

METHOD

STEP 1

Preheat oven to 425ºF. Line a baking sheet with parchment paper. Set aside.

Place butternut squash on a cutting board and using a vegetable peeler, peel your butternut squash.

Once it's peeled, cut your butternut squash in half and remove the seed.

STEP 2

Dice your butternut squash into bite-sized pieces roughly the same size so that they bake evenly.

Place butternut squash on the prepared baking sheet and drizzle on olive oil and season with salt, pepper and paprika.

Toss with your hands and then place in oven.

Roast for 15-20 minutes. Time will depend on the size of the butternut squash cubes.

Garnish with fresh parsley.

NUTRITION VALUE

143 Energy, 5g fat, 1g saturated fat, 5g fiber, 2g protein, 27g carbs.

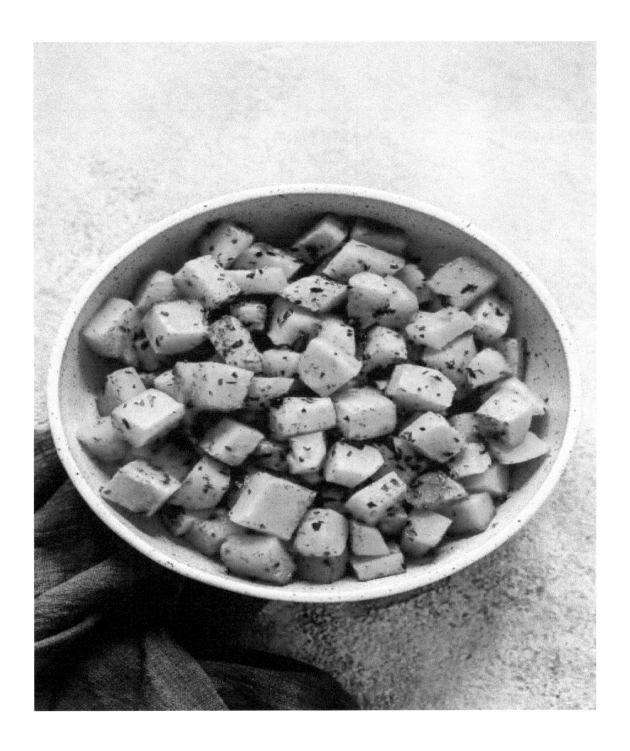

CAULIFLOWER "RICE" TABBOULEH SALAD RECIPE

Cauliflower "Rice" Tabbouleh Salad is an easy low-carb, gluten-free meal that can be prepared in advance making a great "on-the-go" lunch.

MAKES 4 SERVING/ TOTAL TIME 18 MINUTE

INGREDIENTS

1 small cauliflower head - cut off the florets

2 cups cucumber - chopped

2 cups cherry tomatoes - chopped

1 cup fresh parsley - chopped

¼ cup fresh mint - chopped

¼ cup olive oil

2 tablespoons fresh lemon juice

Salt and pepper to taste

METHOD

STEP 1

Pulse the cauliflower florets in a food processor for about 25-30 seconds until it's a rice-like consistency. Place the cauliflower in a microwave-safe bowl and microwave for 3-4 minutes. The time will depend on the power of the microwave.

Once cauliflower is cool enough to handle, transfer to a salad bowl.

STEP 2

Add cucumber, tomatoes, parsley and mint in the salad bowl. In a mason jar, pour the olive oil and freshly squeezed lemon juice. Add salt, pepper and whisk everything together. Continue to whisk while streaming in the olive oil. Taste to check the seasoning.

Pour the dressing over the salad, toss well and enjoy!

NUTRITION VALUE

188 Energy, 15g fat, 2g saturated fat, 5g fiber, 5g protein, 13g carbs.

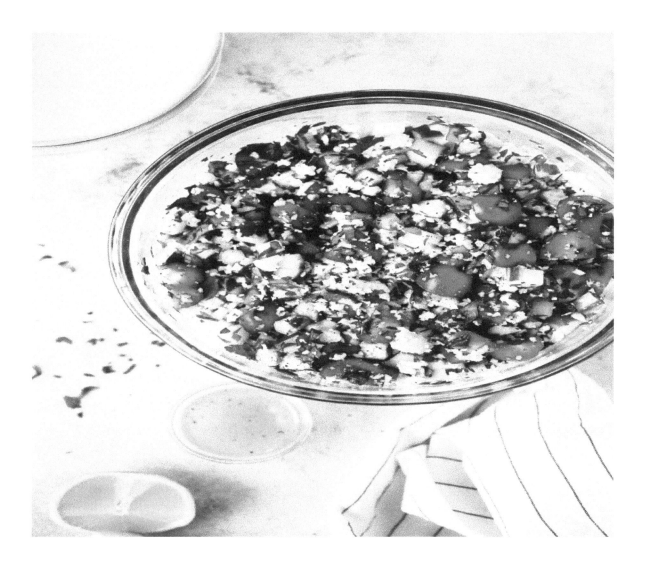

ROASTED RED BELL PEPPER PASTA

This Gluten-free Roasted Red Bell Pepper Pasta is also vegan, made with cashews, roasted red bell pepper, red onions, garlic and almond milk. And it's topped with crispy and super flavorful tofu.

MAKES 6 SERVING/ TOTAL TIME 20 MINUTE

INGREDIENTS

3 red bell peppers - roughly chopped

¼ cup red onions - chopped

1 clove garlic

2 tablespoons olive oil

½ package of Barilla Gluten Free Elbows Pasta

1/2 cup raw cashews

1/2 cup unsweetened almond milk

2 tablespoons nutritional yeast

Salt and black pepper to taste

Red pepper flakes to taste

12 oz. extra firm tofu

Chopped fresh parsley for garnishing

METHOD

STEP 1

Preheat the oven to 450 °F. On a baking sheet lined with parchment paper, mix the red bell peppers, onions, garlic and 1 tablespoon of olive oil and then spread evenly. Bake for 15-20 minutes.

Meanwhile, cook the Barilla Gluten Free Elbows Pasta according to the instructions on the package. Set aside. In a blender or food processor, add the veggies from the oven, raw cashews, milk, nutritional yeast, salt, pepper and red pepper flakes. Blender everything until smooth If you think the texture is too thick you can add more milk according to your taste. Set aside.

STEP 2

Using a paper towel or a clean towel, press the excess moisture out of the tofu. Cut into small square pieces. In a nonstick skillet, heat 1 tablespoon of olive oil.

Add the tofu and stir fry until golden brown. It's about 5-8 minutes. Set aside.

Place the pasta on a plate dish and top with the crispy tofu and fresh chopped parsley. Enjoy!

NUTRITION VALUE

309 Energy, 13.3g fat, 2.3g saturated fat, 4g fiber, 10.7g protein, 41.5g carbs.

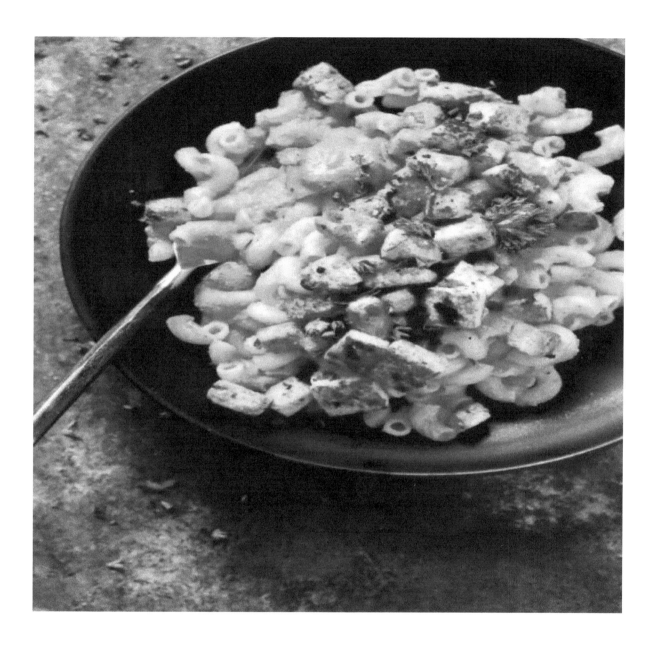

ROASTED BUTTERNUT SQUASH CAULIFLOWER SALAD

You'll love this Roasted Butternut Squash Cauliflower Salad for fall. It's tossed with an easy and very delicious vegan dressing.

MAKES 4 SERVING/ TOTAL TIME 30 MINUTE

INGREDIENTS

FOR THE SALAD

1 medium cauliflower head - cut into florets

1 small butternut squash - peeled and cut in cubes

1 tbsp olive oil

salt and black pepper

¼ cup red onion - chopped

1 tablespoon green onions - chopped

FOR DRESSING

1/2 cup veganaise or traditional mayonnaise

2 tablespoon yellow mustard

1 teaspoon garlic - minced

Salt and pepper

METHOD

STEP 1

First, steam the head of cauliflower. In a large pot add about 2 cups of water and place a steamer basket in the bottom. Bring the water to a boil. Add the cauliflower florets into the steamer basket.

Cover the pot and steam until the cauliflower florets are tender 6-8 minutes. Let the cauliflower cool down for 5 minutes.

STEP 2

Preheat oven to 400 degrees. On a baking sheet lined with parchment paper or silicone mat, place butternut squash and toss in olive oil and season with salt and black pepper. Mix well to combine.

Roast in the oven for 15-20 minutes

Place the steamed cauliflower, the roasted butternut squash and the red onions in a bowl.

In a small glass bowl, add all the ingredients for the dressing and whisk everything together to combine. Taste to check the seasoning and pour over the salad. Mix all the ingredients together until well combined and garnish it with green onions.

NUTRITION VALUE

287 Energy, 22g fat, 1.6g saturated fat, 5.5g fiber, 4g protein, 17.3g carbs.

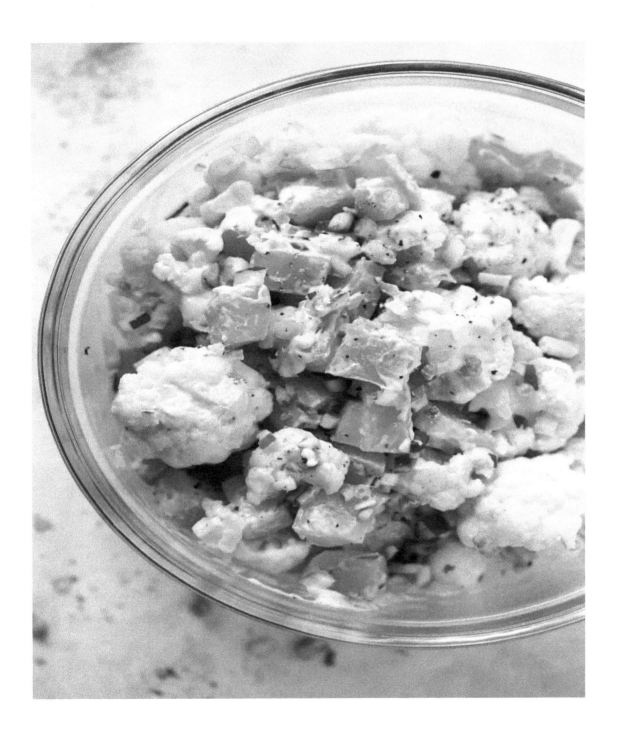

SUGAR SNAP PEA AND CARROT SOBA NOODLES

This recipe yields about six servings and the leftovers don't keep particularly well, so halve the ingredients if you're not serving a crowd.

MAKES 6 SERVING/ TOTAL TIME 30 MINUTE

INGREDIENTS

6 ounces spaghetti noodles of choice

2 cups frozen organic edamame

10 ounces sugar snap peas

6 medium-sized carrots, peeled

½ cup chopped fresh cilantro

¼ cup sesame seeds

Ginger-sesame sauce

¼ cup reduced-sodium tamari

2 tablespoons quality peanut oil

1 tablespoon toasted sesame oil

1 tablespoon honey or agave nectar

2 teaspoons freshly grated ginger

1 teaspoon chili garlic sauce

METHOD

STEP 1

Slice the carrots into long, thin strips with a julienne peeler, or slice them into ribbons with a vegetable peeler. To make the sauce: whisk together the ingredients in a small bowl until emulsified. Set aside. Pour the sesame seeds into a small pan. Toast for about 4 to 5 minutes over medium-low heat, shaking the pan frequently to prevent burning, until the seeds are turning golden and starting to make popping noises.

STEP 2

Once the pots of water are boiling: In one pot, cook the soba noodles just until al dente, according to package directions then drain and briefly rinse under cool water. Cook the frozen edamame in the other pot until warmed through and cook for an additional 20 seconds. Drain. Combine the soba noodles, edamame, snap peas and carrots in a large serving bowl. Pour in the dressing and toss with salad servers. Toss in the chopped cilantro and toasted sesame seeds. Serve.

NUTRITION VALUE

362 Energy, 12.7g fat, 1.6g saturated fat, 4.6g fiber, 17.2g protein, 53g carbs.

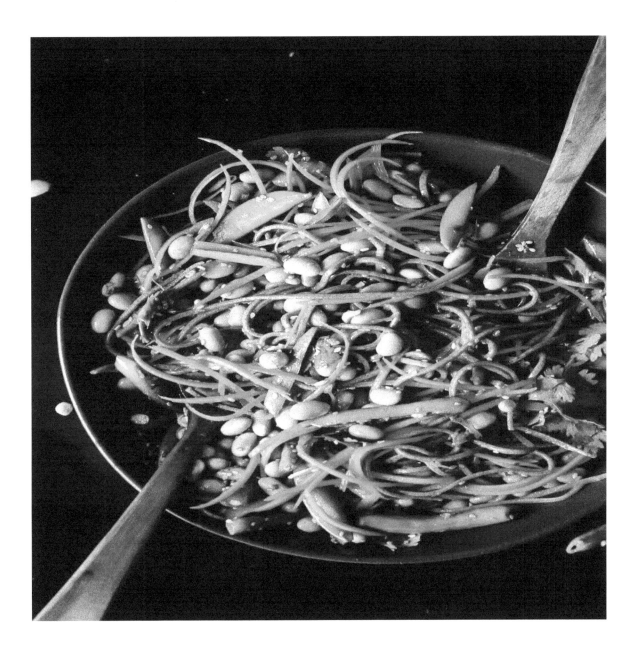

CREAMY (VEGAN!) BUTTERNUT SQUASH LINGUINE WITH FRIED SAGE

Serve with salad or roasted vegetables to further lighten up the meal. Recipe yields 4 large servings.

MAKES 4 SERVING/ TOTAL TIME 55 MINUTE

INGREDIENTS

2 tablespoons olive oil

1 tablespoon finely chopped fresh sage

2-pound butternut or kabocha squash, peeled, seeded, and cut into small ½-inch pieces (about 3 cups)

1 medium yellow onion, chopped

2 garlic cloves, pressed or chopped

⅛ teaspoon red pepper flakes (up to ¼ teaspoon for spicier pasta sauce)

Salt

Freshly ground black pepper

2 cups vegetable broth

12 ounces whole grain linguine

METHOD

STEP 1 Warm the oil in a large skillet over medium heat. Once the oil is shimmering, add the sage and toss to coat Add the squash, onion, garlic and red pepper flakes to the skillet. Season with salt and pepper. Cook, stirring occasionally, until the onion is translucent, about 8 to 10 minutes. Add the broth. Bring the mixture to a boil, then reduce the heat and simmer until the squash is soft and the liquid is reduced by half, about 15 to 20 minutes.

STEP 2

In the meantime, bring a large pot of salted water to a boil and cook the pasta until al dente according to package directions, stirring occasionally. Reserve 1 cup of the pasta cooking water before draining.

Cook over medium heat, tossing and adding more pasta cooking water as needed, until the sauce coats the pasta, about 2 minutes. Season with more salt and pepper if necessary.

Serve the pasta

NUTRITION VALUE	1190 KJ Energy, 8.7g fat, 1.9g saturated fat, 13.6g fiber, 11.3g protein, 32.2g carbs.

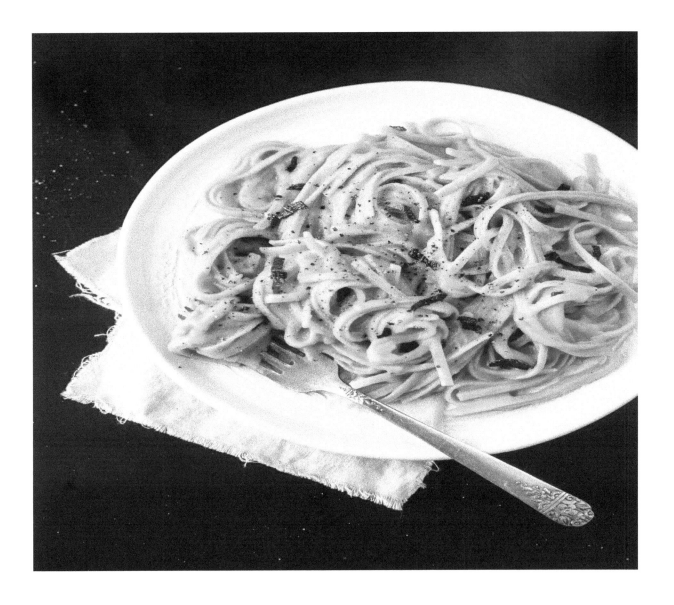

VEGAN SAUSAGE

Vegan sausage, a super convenient and tasty recipe It is 100% plant-based, delicious, and super flavorful, as well as perfect to eat for lunch or dinner!

MAKES 8 SERVING/ TOTAL TIME 1 HOUR 10 MINUTE

INGREDIENTS

1 tbsp extra-virgin olive oil, divided

2 cloves of garlic, sliced

½ onion, chopped

1 14-ounce can cannellini beans

1 tsp fennel seeds

1 tsp dried thyme

1 tsp ground cumin

1 tsp paprika

½ tsp salt

½ tsp ground black pepper

1 tbsp tomato paste

1 tbsp maple syrup

1 tbsp soy sauce or tamari

1 cup vital wheat gluten (120 g)

METHOD

STEP 1

Heat 1 tsp of extra-virgin olive oil in a skillet and cook the garlic and onion over medium-high heat until golden brown, stirring occasionally. Set aside.

Add all the remaining ingredients to a food processor bowl. Then add the cooked garlic and onion and pulse until well combined. Add the vital wheat gluten and pulse again until well combined and it comes together in a ball. It's okay if it's not a perfect ball.

STEP 2

Roll and press the dough into a sausage shape. Roll tightly each sausage in aluminum foil. Twist the ends so that each sausage is completely covered in foil.

Add the vegan sausages into the steaming basket and steam for 40 minutes, flipping them after 20 minutes. Remove from the stove and let them cool for about 5 minutes, then unwrap. Heat the remaining extra-virgin olive oil in a large skillet and then cook the sausages over medium-high heat for about 1 to 2 minutes on each side, You can serve your vegan sausages with BBQ sauce, mustard, vegan mashed potatoes.

NUTRITION VALUE

215 Energy, 2.1g fat, 0.3g saturated fat, 11g fiber, 19.6g protein, 32.2g carbs.

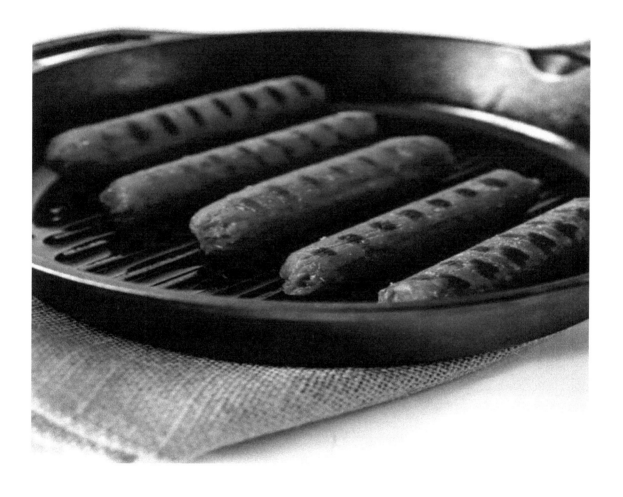

VEGAN POT PIE

Vegan pot pie, one of my favorite comfort recipes ever. It is super warm, cozy, and flavorful, as well as perfect to enjoy during the wintertime.

MAKES 8 SERVING/ TOTAL TIME 1 HOUR

INGREDIENTS

2 batches of vegan pie crust,

2 tbsp vegan butter

3 cloves of garlic, sliced

1 medium onion, chopped

1 celery stick, chopped

2 medium carrots, chopped

12 oz store-bought

⅓ cup all-purpose flour (40 g)

2 cups vegan chicken stock (480 ml),

½ cup unsweetened plant milk

½ cup frozen peas (65 g)

½ tsp salt

¼ tsp ground black pepper

2 tsp dried thyme

2 tbsp fresh parsley, finely chopped

METHOD

STEP 1

Preheat the oven to 400ºF or 200ºC.

Heat the vegan butter (or oil) in a large pot and cook the veggies (garlic, onion, celery, and carrots) over medium-high heat for about 10 minutes or until soft, stirring occasionally. Add the vegan chicken Add the Then add the vegetable stock and the plant milk and stir. After that, incorporate all the remaining ingredients, stir again and cook until it thickens, stirring occasionally.

STEP 2

Pour the filling into the pie crust-lined pan. I use a 9-inch or 23 cm round pie pan.

Roll the second vegan pie crust into a round and place over the pie filling. Fold the excess dough behind the bottom crust then crimp the pie crusts together to seal. Bake for 35 to 45 minutes Remove from the oven and let it rest for 15 minutes to cool slightly before slicing. and serve immediately with breakfast potatoes, roasted red peppers, or your favorite side dish.

NUTRITION VALUE

197 Energy, 8.4g fat, 2g saturated fat, 3g fiber, 9.6g protein, 32.2g carbs.

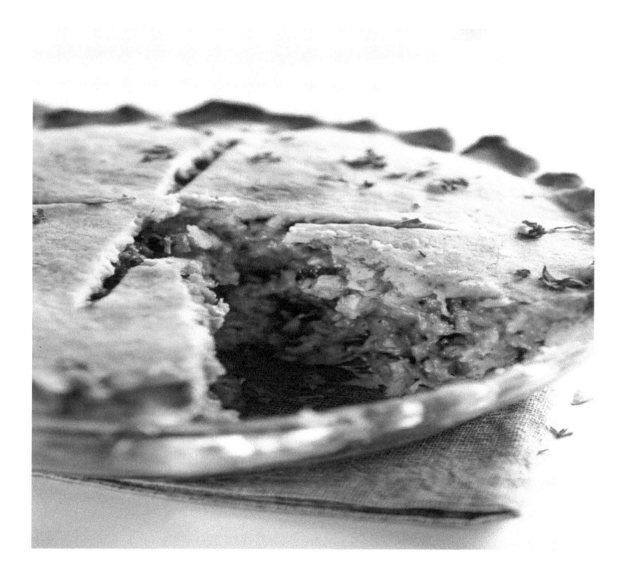

MARINATED TOFU SKEWERS

Recipe that everyone loves!

MAKES 4 SERVING/ TOTAL TIME 2 HOUR

INGREDIENTS

320g Nigari hard tofu, cut into 2.5cm cubes

2 1/2 tablespoons olive oil

2 teaspoons lemon pepper

2 1/2 teaspoons thyme leaves

3 zucchinis, cut into 2cm-thick slices

200g grape tomatoes

12 button mushrooms, halved

200g mixed salad leaves, to serve

4 slices crusty bread, to serve

METHOD

STEP 1
Soak skewers in a shallow dish of cold water for 30 minutes. Drain.

STEP 2
Place tofu, oil, lemon pepper and thyme into a ceramic bowl. Stir to combine. Cover. Refrigerate for 1 hour, if time permits.

STEP 3
Thread tofu, zucchinis tomatoes and mushrooms alternately onto skewers. Brush skewers with remaining marinade mixture.

STEP 4
Preheat a chargrill or barbecue grill on high heat. Reduce heat to medium. Cook skewers for 5 to 6 minutes, turning occasionally, or until vegetables and tofu are lightly charred and just tender.

STEP 5
Divide salad between serving plates. Top with skewers. Serve with bread.

NUTRITION VALUE

1135 KJ Energy, 17.9g fat, 2.5g saturated fat, 5.8g fiber, 14.1g protein, 13.6g carbs.

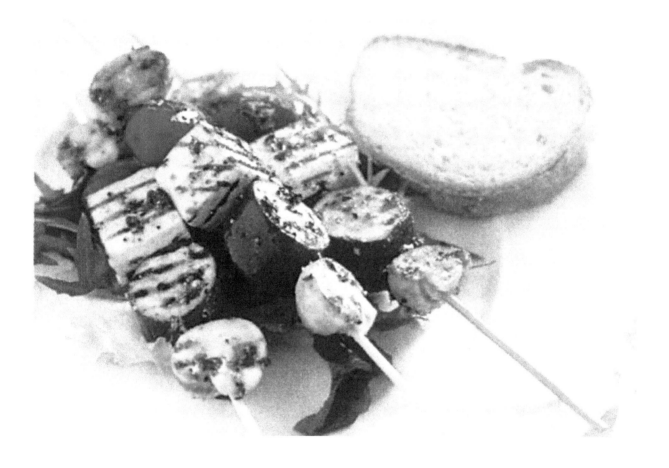

ASPARAGUS WITH CHILLI PANGRATTATO

Blanch green asparagus spears until tender crisp, then shower with herbed breadcrumbs for a super-healthy side.

MAKES 6 SERVING/ TOTAL TIME 25 MINUTE

INGREDIENTS

100g crusty bread

1 long fresh red chili, halved, deseeded, coarsely chopped

Olive oil spray

3 bunches asparagus woody ends trimmed

2 tablespoons chopped fresh continental parsley

Lemon wedges, to serve

METHOD

STEP 1

Remove the crusts from the bread and discard. Coarsely chop the bread. Place the bread and chili in the bowl of a food processor and process until finely chopped.

STEP 2

Place the bread mixture in a non-stick frying pan over low heat. Spray with olive oil spray. Cook, stirring occasionally, for 6-8 minutes or until crisp and golden.

STEP 3

Bring a large, deep frying pan of water to the boil over high heat. Add the asparagus and cook for 2 minutes or until bright green and tender crisp. Refresh under cold running water. Drain.

STEP 4

Add the parsley to the bread mixture and stir to combine. Transfer the asparagus to a serving platter and sprinkle with the bread mixture. Serve with lemon wedges.

NUTRITION VALUE

290 KJ Energy, 1g fat, 2.5g fiber, 4.5g protein, 11g carbs.

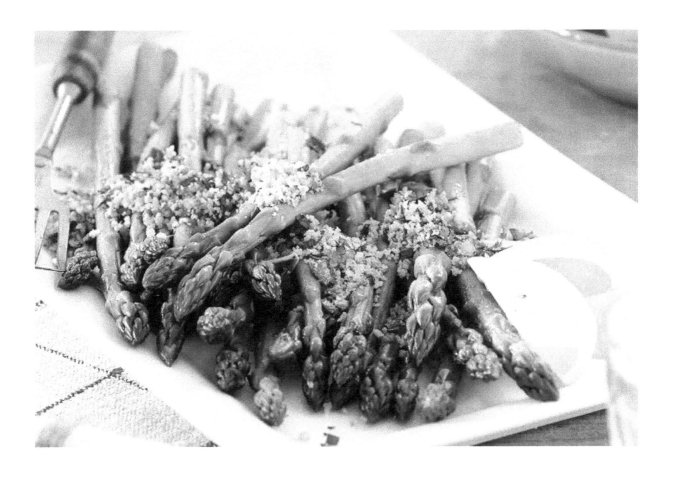

PUMPKIN AND CHICKPEA SALAD

This pumpkin and chickpea salad recipe is vegan friendly.

MAKES 6 SERVING/ TOTAL TIME 35 MINUTE

INGREDIENTS

1.2kg butternut pumpkin, peeled, deseeded, cut into 2cm pieces

1/3 cup olive oil

1 teaspoon ground coriander

1 teaspoon ground cumin

400g can Coles Chickpeas, drained, rinsed

6 dessert figs, finely chopped (see note)

1 small red onion, halved, thinly sliced

1/2 cup coriander leaves, roughly chopped

1 large lemon, rind grated, juiced

Salt, to season

METHOD

STEP 1

Preheat oven to 200°C. Lightly grease a large roasting pan. Combine pumpkin, 2 tablespoons oil, ground coriander and cumin in a large bowl. Season with salt and pepper. Transfer to prepared pan. Roast for 20 minutes or until pumpkin is tender. Allow to cool.

STEP 2

Combine pumpkin, chickpeas, figs, onion and chopped coriander in a large bowl.

STEP 3

Combine remaining 2 tablespoons oil, lemon rind, 2 tablespoons lemon juice and salt and pepper in a jug. Pour over pumpkin. Toss until well combined. Serve.

NUTRITION VALUE

1126 KJ Energy, 14g fat, 2g saturated fat, 6g protein, 24g carbs.

70

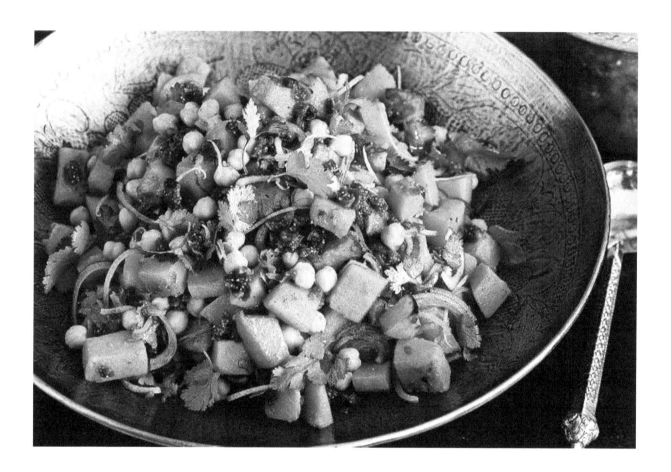

ASIAN GREENS AND TOFU SALAD

Asian greens tossed with tofu makes a quick and simple quick accompaniment to an oriental inspired feast.

MAKES 12 SERVING/ TOTAL TIME 30 MINUTE

INGREDIENTS

3 bunches (about 840g) snake beans, cut into 7cm lengths

2 bunches (about 500g) baby book choy, quartered lengthways, washed

1 bunch coriander, leaves picked

2 300g pkts firm tofu, drained, cut crossways into 1cm-thick slices

250ml (1 cup) peanut oil

100ml soy sauce

5cm piece fresh ginger, peeled, finely grated

METHOD

STEP 1

Cook the snake beans in a large saucepan of salted boiling water for 2-3 minutes or until bright green and tender crisp. Cook the bok choy in the same saucepan of salted boiling water for 1 minute. Drain and refresh under cold running water. Combine the snake beans, baby bok choy and coriander in a large bowl and gently toss until combined.

STEP 2

Place the tofu in a single layer in a large shallow glass or ceramic dish. Whisk together the peanut oil, soy sauce and ginger in a small bowl. Spoon the marinade over the tofu. Cover with plastic wrap and place in the fridge for 1 hour to marinate. Cook the tofu on preheated barbecue grill or chargrill for 2 minutes each side or until browned and heated through.

STEP 3

Place the snake bean mixture in a large serving bowl and drizzle with half the reserved marinade. Gently toss to combine.

NUTRITION VALUE

1120 KJ Energy, 23g fat, 7g saturated fat, 4g fiber, 10g protein, 3g carbs.

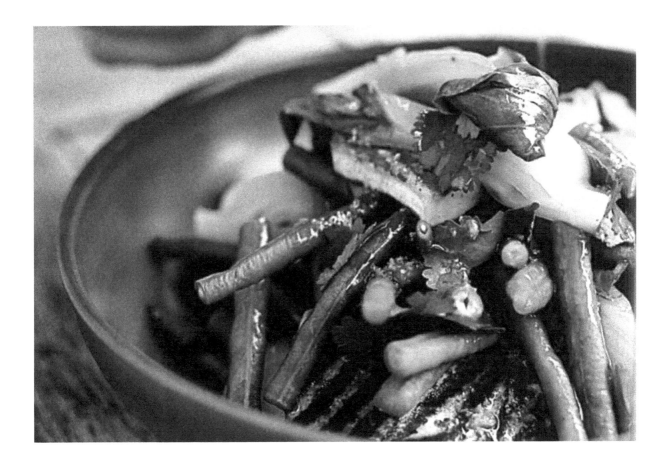

MUSHROOM RICE PAPER ROLLS

Start off your Asian-inspired feast with these mushroom rice paper rolls.

MAKES 4 SERVING/ TOTAL TIME 23 MINUTE

INGREDIENTS

1 tablespoon sesame oil

2 cloves garlic, crushed

1 teaspoon grated ginger

2 shallots, finely diced

300g button mushrooms, chopped

40g Chinese cabbage, finely shredded

2 teaspoons low-salt soy sauce

16 large sheets of rice paper

1 bunch fresh coriander, leaves picked

2 medium carrots, peeled, finely julienned

1 cup bean sprouts, trimmed

Extra low-salt soy sauce, to serve

METHOD

STEP 1

Heat sesame oil, garlic, and ginger in a frying pan and over low heat for 1 minute. Add shallots, mushrooms, and cabbage and increase heat to medium. Cook for 3 minutes or until just tender. Transfer to a bowl, add soy and set aside to cool.

STEP 2

Fill a large bowl with warm water, and place 2 rice paper sheets at a time into the water to soften for about 30 seconds. Be careful not to let them get too soft - they should be soft, but firm enough to handle.

STEP 3

Remove rice paper from water, and drain well and lay on a flat board. Sprinkle with coriander leaves and sandwich with the second sheet of rice paper. Top with a tablespoon of mushroom mixture (be careful to drain excess moisture). Top with julienned carrot and bean sprouts. Fold the ends in and roll up firmly. Set aside and cover with plastic. Continue with remaining ingredients. Serve immediately.

NUTRITION VALUE

1060 KJ Energy, 5.5g fat, 1g saturated fat, 45g carbs.

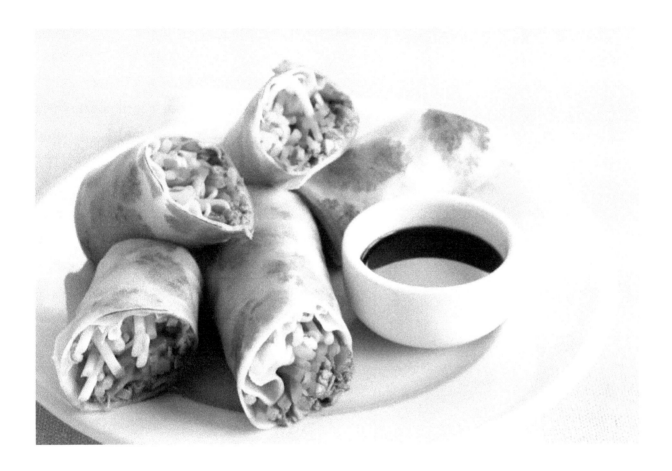

HASSELBACK POTATOES

Recipe that everyone loves!

MAKES 8 SERVING/ TOTAL TIME 1 HOUR 20 MINUTE

INGREDIENTS

12 medium Pontiac potatoes, peeled, halved

1 tablespoon olive oil

2 tablespoons finely chopped fresh flat-leaf parsley leaves

2 tablespoons finely chopped fresh oregano leaves

1/4 cup dried breadcrumbs

METHOD

STEP 1

Preheat oven to 200°C/180°C fan-forced. Place potato, cut side down on a chopping board. Using a sharp knife, make small vertical cuts through each potato (being careful not to cut all the way through). Place potatoes in a large roasting pan.

STEP 2

Add oil, parsley, oregano and breadcrumbs to pan. Season with salt and pepper. Toss to combine. Roast potatoes for 1 hour or until golden and tender.

NUTRITION VALUE

740 KJ Energy, 2.6g fat, 0.4g saturated fat, 4.2g fiber, 5.5g protein, 29.8g carbs.

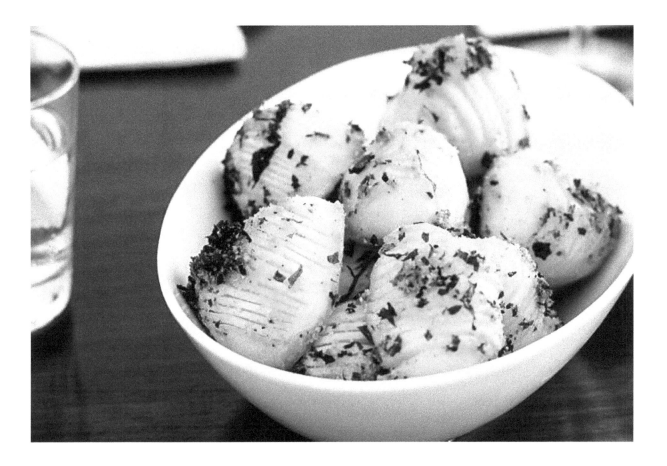

BROCCOLI AND LENTIL SALAD WITH CHILLI AND PINE NUTS

Infused with balsamic vinegar, this easy salad is delicious as well as super healthy.

MAKES 4 SERVING/ TOTAL TIME 27 MINUTE

INGREDIENTS

600g broccoli trimmed, cut into florets

1 x 400g can brown lentils, rinsed, drained

2 teaspoons balsamic vinegar

1 tablespoon olive oil

6 shallots, ends trimmed, thinly sliced

1 long fresh red chili, deseeded, finely chopped

2 garlic cloves, thinly sliced

75g baby spinach leaves

2 tablespoons toasted pine nuts

METHOD

STEP 1

Cook the broccoli in a large saucepan of boiling water for 3-4 minutes or until bright green and tender crisp. Refresh under cold running water. Drain.

STEP 2

Place the lentils in a bowl. Whisk together the vinegar and 2 teaspoons of olive oil. Add to lentils. Stir to combine.

STEP 3

Heat the remaining oil in a large non-stick frying pan over medium heat. Add the shallot, chili and garlic. Cook, stirring, for 1 minute or until aromatic. Add the broccoli and cook, stirring occasionally, for 2 minutes or until heated through and the broccoli is coated in the shallot mixture.

STEP 4

Add the broccoli mixture and spinach to the lentil mixture. Season with pepper. Toss to combine.

STEP 5

Sprinkle with the pine nuts to serve.

NUTRITION VALUE

796 KJ Energy, 11g fat, 1g saturated fat, 9g fiber, 12g protein, 7g carbs.

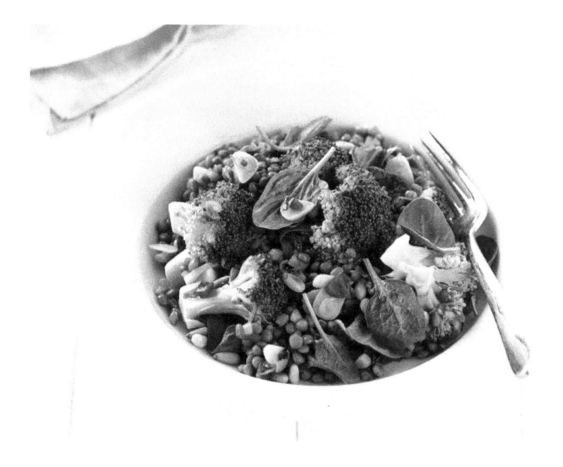

POTATO, MINT & OLIVE SALAD

Mint and olive liven up this summer potato salad.

MAKES 10 SERVING/ TOTAL TIME 30 MINUTE

INGREDIENTS

20 chat (small coli ban) potatoes, halved

145g (1 cup) drained pitted kalamata olives, coarsely chopped

1 cup loosely packed fresh mint leaves, coarsely chopped

2 tablespoons coarsely chopped fresh continental parsley

60ml (1/4 cup) olive oil

2 teaspoons sea salt flakes

METHOD

STEP 1

Place potato in a large saucepan and cover with cold water. Cover with a lid and bring to the boil over high heat. Boil for 8 minutes or until tender. Drain and set aside for 1 hour or until cool.

STEP 2

Place potato in a large serving bowl. Add the olives, mint, parsley, oil and sea salt flakes, and gently toss to combine.

NUTRITION VALUE

776 KJ Energy, 4 fat, 1g saturated fat, 4g protein, 24g carbs.

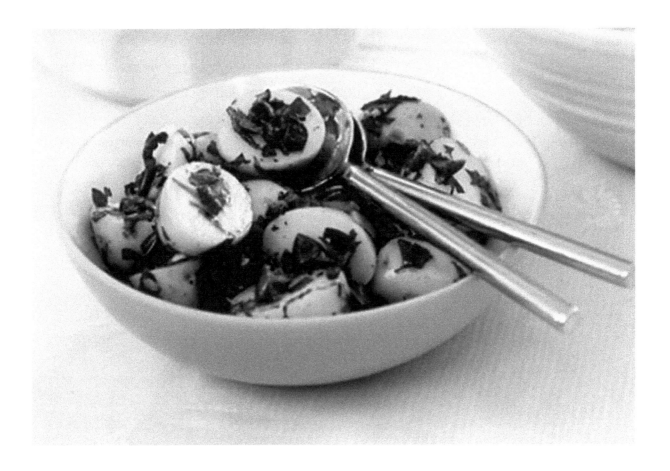

PIMIENTOS DE PADRON

Recipe that everyone loves!

MAKES 10 SERVING/ TOTAL TIME 10 MINUTE

INGREDIENTS

2 tablespoons olive oil

300g green pimientos de Padron chilies (Spanish green chilies)

1/2 cup (80g) raw almonds

METHOD
STEP 1

Heat the oil in a large fry pan over medium-high heat. Add the pimientos and cook for 3-4 minutes until the skins begin to char. Add nuts and a tablespoon of sea salt, and stir for 1 minute to heat through. Serve warm and beware!

NUTRITION VALUE

363 KJ Energy, 8 g fat, 1g saturated fat, 2g protein, 1g carbs.

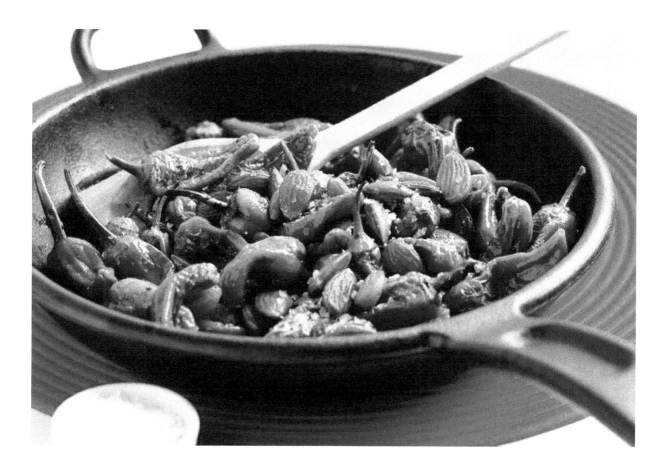

VEGETABLE SUNG CHOI BAO

Recipe that everyone loves!

MAKES 4 SERVING/ TOTAL TIME 15 MINUTE

INGREDIENTS

1 425g can young corn cuts, drained

1 280g can mushrooms, drained

1 230g can water chestnuts, drained

3 green shallots, trimmed, chopped

2 teaspoons olive oil

1 garlic clove, crushed

3 teaspoons soy sauce

1 teaspoon finely chopped fresh ginger

4 whole iceberg lettuce inner leaves, washed, dried

Coriander leaves, to serve

METHOD

STEP 1

Place the corn, mushrooms, water chestnuts and green shallots in the bowl of a food processor. Process until roughly chopped.

STEP 2

Heat the oil in a wok or medium non-stick frying pan over medium-high heat. Add the vegetable mixture, garlic, soy sauce and ginger, and stir-fry for 2-3 minutes or until heated through.

STEP 3

Divide the mixture among the lettuce cups. Sprinkle with the coriander leaves and serve immediately.

NUTRITION VALUE

223 KJ Energy, 3g fat,
6g fiber, 3g protein, 2g carbs.

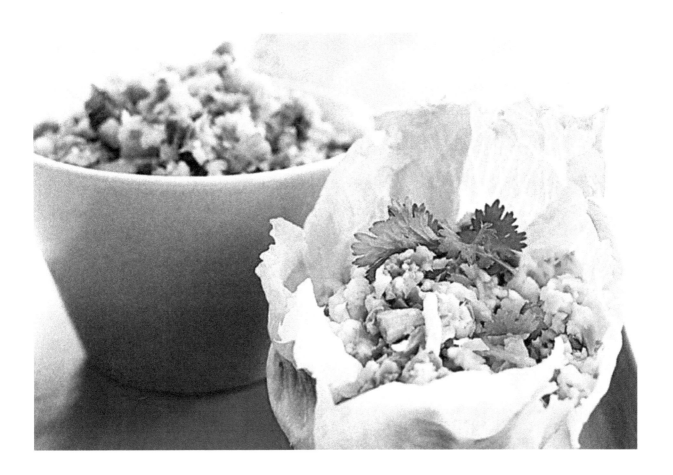

VEGAN TUNA SANDWICH

This vegan tuna sandwich is ready in less than 10 minutes. It's a delicious, simple and healthy lunch recipe, perfect to bring to work or school.

MAKES 4 SERVING/ TOTAL TIME 10 MINUTE

INGREDIENTS

For the vegan tuna:

7 ounces canned or cooked chickpeas

1/4 cup tahini (4 tbsp)

2 tbsp lemon juice

2 tbsp yellow mustard

1 tbsp nori flakes (optional)

1/4 chopped red onion

4 vinegar pickles (1 oz or 30 g)

1/2 chopped celery stalk

1/4 tsp salt

1/8 tsp ground black pepper

For the sandwich:

8 whole wheat bread slices

Lettuce leaves

2 sliced tomatoes

METHOD

STEP 1

Place all the vegan tuna ingredients in a food processor or blender and blend until you get a thick spread, as you can see in the third picture.

Toast the bread in a toaster, frying pan or panini press. Place the lettuce leaves onto four pieces of bread, then the vegan tuna and finally the tomato slices. Top with the other four slices of bread.

This sandwich is better fresh, although it's also a great lunch recipe to bring to work or school.

Store the vegan tuna in a sealed container in the fridge for up to 4 days.

NUTRITION VALUE

317 Energy, 11.7g fat, 1.7g saturated fat, 8.7g fiber, 14g protein, 41.6g carbs.

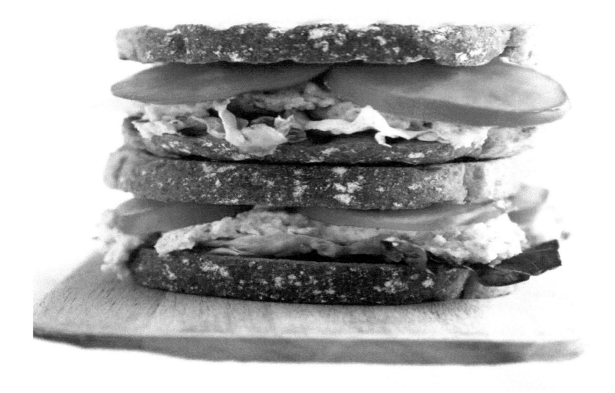

VEGAN BURRITO BOWL

This burrito bowl is so tasty and satisfying. It's also a great way to use up leftovers and it can also be a great lunch box recipe.

MAKES 2 SERVING/ TOTAL TIME 30 MINUTE

INGREDIENTS

1/2 cup short-grain white rice, uncooked (100 g)

1/2 cup frozen corn kernels (80 g)

Fat-free vegan refried beans

1 cup red cabbage, julienned (100 g)

4 romaine lettuce leaves, julienned

1 sliced avocado

1 chopped tomato

A handful of fresh tomato, finely chopped

Tahini salad dressing to taste

METHOD

STEP 1

Cook the rice and the corn kernels, according to package directions. We don't add any salt.

Prepare the fat-free vegan refried beans. Use our recipe if you want.

To assemble the burrito bowl just place the rice, refried beans, red cabbage and lettuce in the bowl and garnish with the rest of the ingredients.

Add dressing to taste and serve.

NUTRITION VALUE

295 Energy, 8.6g fat, 1.3g saturated fat, 9.8g fiber, 9g protein, 47.8g carbs.

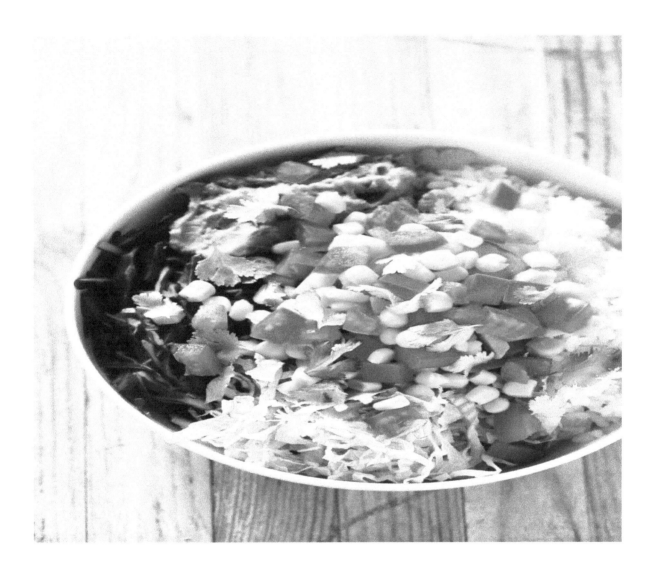

VEGAN BAGEL SANDWICH

This vegan bagel sandwich is ready in less than 10 minutes and is perfect if you want something delicious, quick and easy to make.

MAKES 2 SERVING/ TOTAL TIME 10 MINUTE

INGREDIENTS

2 bagels

8 pitted black olives

1/2 cup vegan cream cheese (100 g)

12 basil leaves

10 sun-dried tomatoes

METHOD

STEP 1

Toast split bagel halves until golden brown.

Chop the olives and place them in a bowl with the cream cheese. Mix until well combined.

STEP 2

Spread the cheese over the bottom halves of each bagel and add the basil leaves and the tomatoes.

Top with remaining bagel halves to make sandwiches.

NUTRITION VALUE

464 Energy, 21.3g fat, 6.5g saturated fat, 6.3g fiber, 14.6g protein, 59.3g carbs.

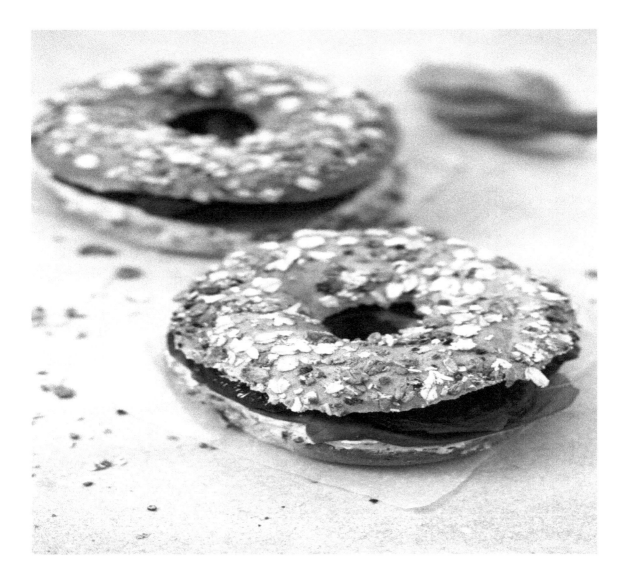

VEGAN SPANISH TOFU SCRAMBLE WITH POTATOES AND CHORIZO

You won't believe this vegan Spanish tofu scramble with potatoes and chorizo is vegan.

MAKES 4 SERVING/ TOTAL TIME 40 MINUTE

INGREDIENTS

Extra-virgin olive oil

¾ cup vegan chopped chorizo (100 g)

½ onion

2 medium potatoes

9.7 oz tofu (275 g)

⅛ tsp turmeric powder (optional)

Sea salt and black pepper to taste

Dash of black salt or Kala Namak (optional)

METHOD

STEP 1

Heat a little bit of extra-virgin olive oil in a frying pan over medium heat and when it's hot, cook the vegan chorizo (chopped) until it starts to golden brown. Set aside. Peel the potatoes and wash them. Cut them in half lengthwise. Then, slice the potatoes in pieces approximately 3 mm or ⅛" thick. Peel and chop the onion into small pieces.

STEP 2

In a non-stick frying pan, place one or two tablespoons of olive oil and when it's hot, add the potatoes, onion, salt to taste and 250 milliliters Cook for about 15 or 20 minutes or until potatoes are soft. Stir occasionally. Add more water if it's necessary. Remove the potatoes and onion from the pan with a slotted spoon. Set aside. Add the turmeric powder, sea salt , black pepper, black salt and cooked chorizo, potatoes and onion. Cook for about 5 minutes.

NUTRITION VALUE

212 Energy, 10.6g fat, 1.1g saturated fat, 8.9g fiber, 10.8g protein, 21.5g carbs.

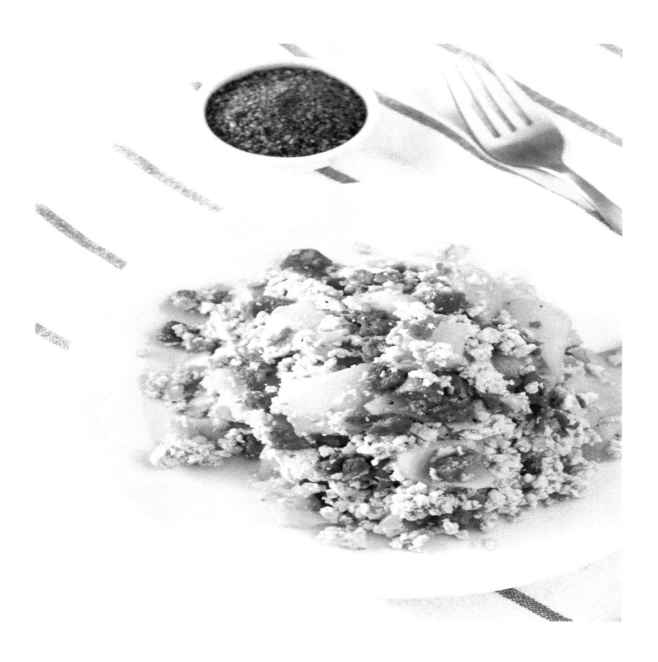

MARINATED TOFU

Marinated tofu, a super simple recipe that makes tofu taste amazing. It's low in fat, high in protein, and only requires 8 ingredients and 20 minutes.

MAKES 2 SERVING/ TOTAL TIME 20 MINUTE

INGREDIENTS

12 oz firm tofu (340 g), cubed

1/4 cup water (60 ml)

2 tbsp soy sauce or tamari

1 tbsp apple cider vinegar

1 tbsp maple syrup

1 tsp garlic powder

1/8 tsp cayenne powder

1 tsp cornstarch

1 tbsp extra-virgin olive oil

METHOD

STEP 1

Mix all the tofu marinade ingredients in a mixing bowl (water, soy sauce, vinegar, syrup, garlic powder, and cayenne powder) until well combined. Add the tofu cubes and let them marinate covered in the fridge for a least 15 minutes. If you let them marinate for a longer period of time, they will have a more intense flavor. Drain the tofu but don't discard the liquid. Set aside. Heat the oil in a skillet and sauté the tofu over medium-high heat until golden brown, stirring occasionally.

STEP 2

Add the marinade liquid to a bowl with the cornstarch and mix until well combined. Pour the sauce into the frying pan and cook until it thickens.

Serve immediately (I added some chopped chives on top, but this is completely optional).

NUTRITION VALUE

145 Energy, 5.8g fat, 1.2g saturated fat, 1.6g fiber, 13.4g protein, 12.4g carbs.

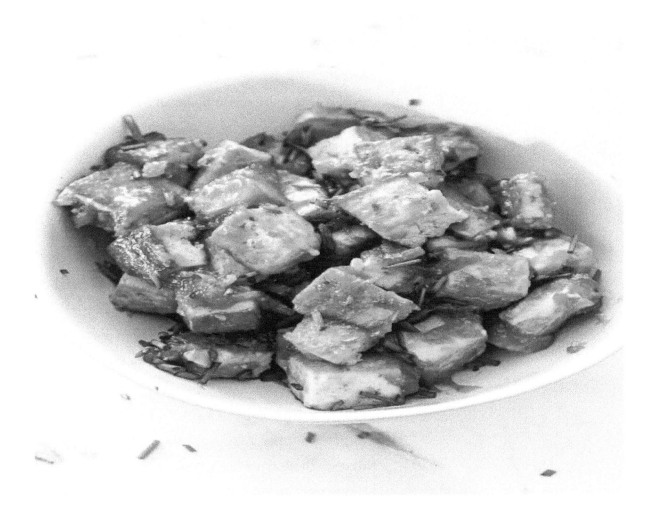

BLACK BEAN BURGERS

Black bean burgers, flavorful, oil and gluten-free, low in fat, and high in fiber and protein. They're ready in just 30 minutes with only 9 ingredients!

MAKES 4 SERVING/ TOTAL TIME 30 MINUTE

INGREDIENTS

2 cups canned or cooked black beans (380 g)

1 and 1/2 cups oats (120 g), I used quick oats, gluten-free if needed

1/4 cup nutritional yeast (4 tbsp)

2 tbsp ground flax seeds

1 tbsp tamari or soy sauce

1 tbsp onion powder

1 tbsp garlic powder

2 tsp paprika

2 tsp cumin powder

METHOD

STEP 1

Feel free to use canned beans or cook them from scratch. If you're going to cook them, use 1 cup of dried black beans (190 g). Drain and wash your canned beans. If you're using cooked beans, you just need to drain them.

STEP 2

Add canned or cooked beans to a large mixing bowl and mash them. I prefer to use an immersion blender, but a fork or a potato masher is also okay.

Add all the remaining ingredients and mash again until well combined. Add more oats if needed.

Make 4 or 5 patties with your hands.

I usually cook them on a griddle for about 5 to 10 minutes or until golden brown with no oil, but feel free to cook them with some oil if you want to.

Enjoy by themselves or serve them with some bread or toppings like tahini, ketchup, tomato slices, and lettuce.

NUTRITION VALUE	188 Energy, 3g fat, 0.3g saturated fat, 10.9g fiber, 12.9g protein, 29.7g carbs.

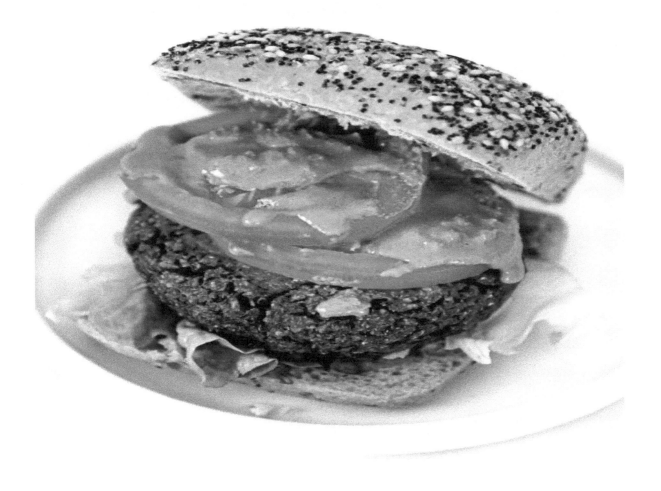

VEGETABLE CURRY

Vegetable curry, a tasty and satiating dish, made with sweet potatoes and veggies, among other ingredients. It's super comforting and nutritious!

MAKES 4 SERVING/ TOTAL TIME 40 MINUTE

INGREDIENTS

1–2 tbsp extra-virgin olive oil

2 cloves of garlic, sliced

1/2 onion, chopped

1/2-inch piece of ginger root

1 zucchini, chopped

1/2 head of cauliflower, chopped,

2 tsp curry powder

1/2 tsp salt

1-pound sweet potatoes (450 g),

1/4 cup tomato paste (4 tbsp or 65 ml)

1 14-ounce can of full-fat coconut milk

1 cup vegetable stock

3 cups baby spinach

METHOD

STEP 1

Heat the oil in a large pot and cook the garlic, onion, an ginger over medium-high heat for 5 minutes, stirring occasionally.

Add the zucchinis and cauliflower and cook for 5 minutes, stirring occasionally.

Add the spices stir, and cook for 1 to 2 minutes, stirring frequently.

STEP 2

Incorporate the sweet potatoes, tomato paste, coconut milk, and vegetable stock, stir, and bring to a boil.

Partially cover and simmer for 15 minutes or until the sweet potatoes are tender.

Add the baby spinach, uncover, stir, and cook for 2 to 3 minutes.

Remove from the stove, add the lemon juice and coconut flour, stir, and let it stand for 5 minutes before serving.

Serve with vegan meat like seitan or tempeh.

NUTRITION VALUE	437 Energy, 23.8g fat, 18.1g saturated fat, 11.4g fiber, 7.6g protein, 51.6g carbs.

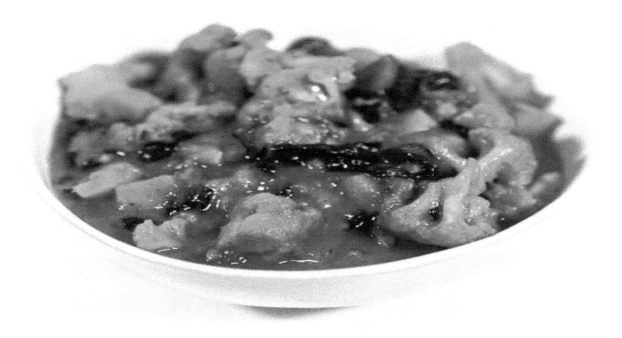

PASTA AGLIO E OLIO

Pasta aglio and olio (known as spaghetti aglio and olio) is the easiest pasta recipe you can make. It's super tasty and only requires 5 ingredients.

MAKES 2 SERVING/ TOTAL TIME 15 MINUTE

INGREDIENTS

1 pound spaghetti (225 g or 16 oz), gluten-free if needed

4 cloves of garlic, sliced

1/4 cup extra-virgin olive oil (4 tbsp)

Dash of red pepper flakes (optional)

1 tbsp fresh parsley, finely chopped

METHOD

STEP 1

Bring a large pot of salted water to the boil and cook the spaghetti according to package directions.

In the meanwhile, add the garlic and oil to a skillet and cook over medium heat until golden brown, stirring occasionally. Add the red pepper flakes and cook for 1-2 minutes more.

STEP 2

Drain the pasta and place it back to the pot, add the oil mixture and the parsley. Toss until the pasta is evenly coated. Add more oil or some cooking water if the pasta is too dry for you.

Serve immediately or keep leftovers in an airtight container in the fridge for 3-4 days.

NUTRITION VALUE

334 Energy, 14.9g fat, 2.2g saturated fat, 1.9g fiber, 7.6g protein, 43.1g carbs.

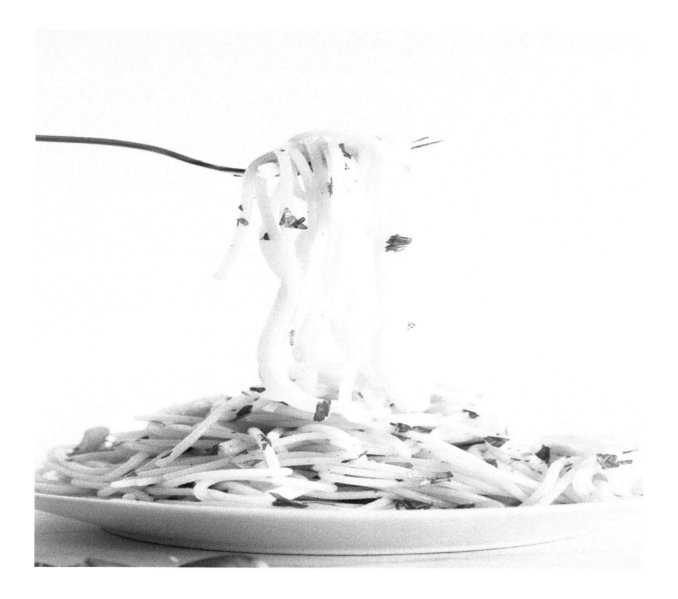

15 MINUTE COCONUT GREEN PASTA

15-minute coconut green pasta. You're going to love this recipe, it's quick, easy, creamy, exotic, spicy, tasty and so delicious! Only 9 ingredients needed!

MAKES 14 SERVING/ TOTAL TIME 15 MINUTE

INGREDIENTS

14 oz gluten-free pasta (400 grams)

1 teaspoon extra-virgin olive oil

4 cloves of garlic

1 cayenne pepper or 1 tsp chili powder

13.5 fl ounces coconut milk (400 milliliters)

1 tbsp lemon juice

1 teaspoon ground ginger

Black pepper to taste

2 cups spinach (60 grams)

METHOD

STEP 1

Cook the minced garlic and the cayenne pepper (chopped) with olive oil until golden brown.
Add the coconut milk, lemon juice, ground ginger and pepper and cook over medium heat for at least 5 minutes.

STEP 2

Transfer to a blender and add the spinach. Blend until smooth. Cook the pasta according to package directions. Drain the pasta and pour it into the pan with the sauce and mix them. You can cook both for 5 minutes more for a more intense flavor.

NUTRITION VALUE

579 Energy, 23.1g fat, 18.5g saturated fat, 3.7g fiber, 15.7g protein, 79.4g carbs.

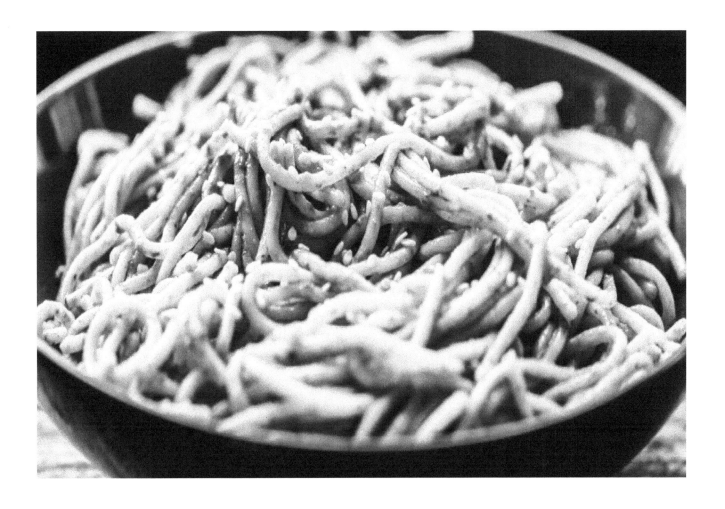

LENTIL SPAGHETTI BOLOGNAISE

Lentils are a healthy and budget friendly alternative to meat bolognaise.

MAKES 6 SERVING/ TOTAL TIME 45 MINUTE

INGREDIENTS

1 tablespoon olive oil

1 brown onion, finely chopped

2 celery sticks, ends trimmed, finely chopped

2 carrots, peeled, coarsely grated

2 garlic cloves, crushed

115g dried split red lentils

1 x 400g can chopped tomatoes

500ml (2 cups) Massel vegetable liquid stock

2 tablespoons tomato paste

500g spaghetti

METHOD

STEP 1

Heat the oil in a large saucepan over medium heat. Add the onion, celery, carrot and garlic, and cook, stirring, for 4 minutes or until the vegetables soften.

STEP 2

Stir in the lentils, tomato, stock and tomato paste. Season with salt and pepper. Increase heat to medium-high and bring to the boil. Reduce heat to medium. Simmer, partially covered, for 20 minutes or until the mixture thickens.

STEP 3

Meanwhile, cook the pasta in a large saucepan of salted boiling water following packet directions or until al dente. Drain and return to the pan.

STEP 4

Add sauce to pasta. Combine. Serve.

NUTRITION VALUE

1736 KJ Energy, 5g fat, 1g saturated fat, 8g fiber, 16g protein, 71g carbs.

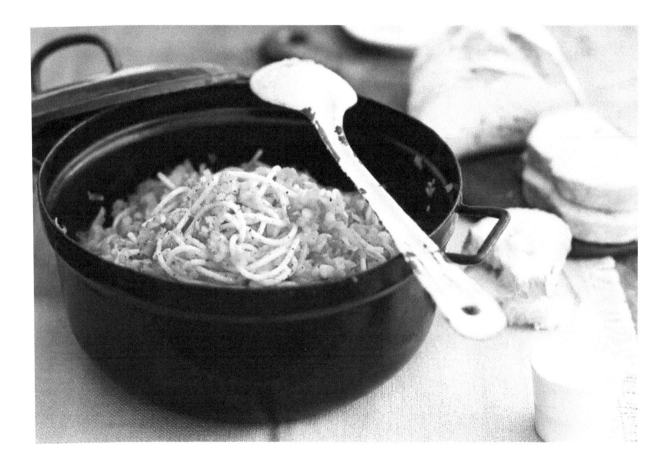

STEP-BY-STEP GNOCCHI

If you've always wondered how to make gnocchi from scratch, these step-by-step gnocchi recipe explains everything you need to know. Just add your favorite sauce and voila!

MAKES 4 SERVING/ TOTAL TIME 1 HOUR 20 MINUTE

INGREDIENTS

4 (750g) desiree potatoes, unpeeled

1 1/3 cups (200g) plain flour, plus a little extra

METHOD

STEP 1

Place potatoes in a saucepan. Cover with cold water and bring to the boil over high heat. Cook for 20-25 minutes or until just tender when tested with a skewer . Drain well. Add flour to potatoes then use your hands to knead briefly until a soft dough form. Cut dough into 4 equal-sized pieces. Using your hands, gently roll each piece out to form a log about 2cm wide. Using a lightly floured knife, cut each log into 1.5cm-long pieces.

STEP 2

Roll each ball of gnocchi over the tines of a lightly-floured fork, pressing gently with your index finger or thumb underneath as you go, to form a dent in the back of each one and fork marks on the other side.

STEP 3

Bring a large saucepan of water to the boil. Add 1/4 of the gnocchi. As they cook, gnocchi will rise to the surface of the water. Continue cooking gnocchi at the surface for about 10 seconds then remove with a large slotted spoon and drain well.

NUTRITION VALUE

1197 KJ Energy, 1g fat, 5g fiber, 10g protein, 57g carbs.

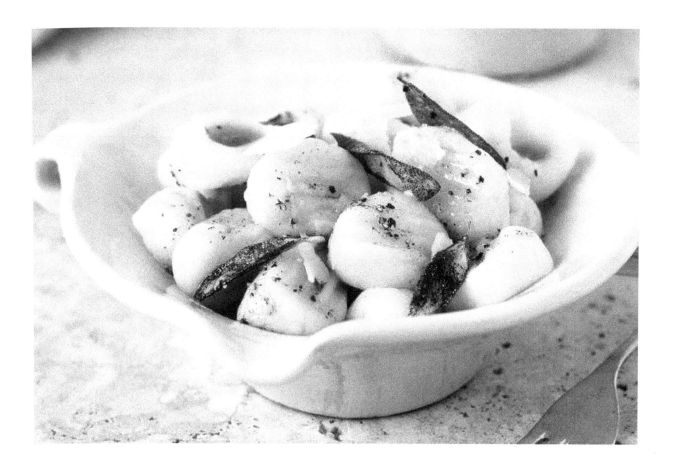

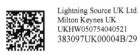